Handbook of PEDIATRIC PHYSICAL THERAPY

Handbook of PEDIATRIC PHYSICAL THERAPY

Toby M. Long, Ph.D., P.T.
Assistant Professor
Department of Physical Therapy
University of Maryland at Baltimore
Baltimore, Maryland
Director, Division of Physical Therapy
Child Development
Georgetown University
Washington, D.C.

Holly Lea Cintas, Ph.D., P.T., P.C.S.
Physical Therapy Research Coordinator
Rehabilitation Medicine Department
National Institutes of Health
Bethesda, Maryland
Past President
Section on Pediatrics
American Physical Therapy Association

SANS TACHE

Williams & Wilkins
BALTIMORE • PHILADELPHIA • HONG KONG
LONDON • MUNICH • SYDNEY • TOKYO
A WAVERLY COMPANY

ISBN 0-683-05155-5

Editor: John P. Butler
Managing Editor: Linda S. Napora
Copy Editor: Julia Robertson Acker
Designer: Wilma E. Rosenberger
Illustration Planner: Wayne Hubbel
Production Coordinator: Anne G. Seitz

Williams & Wilkins
428 East Preston Street
Baltimore, Maryland 21202, USA

Accurate indications, adverse reactions, and dosage schedules for drugs are provided in this book, but it is possible that they may change. The reader is urged to review the package information data of the manufacturers of the medications mentioned.

Printed in the United States of America

Library of Congress Cataloging-in-Publication Data

Long, Toby M.
Handbook of pediatric physical therapy / Toby M. Long, Holly Lea Cintas.
p. cm.
Includes bibliographical references and index.
ISBN 0-683-05155-5
1. Physical therapy for children. I. Cintas, Holly Lea II. Title.
[DNLM: 1. Physical Therapy—in infancy & childhood. 2. Child Development Disorders—therapy. WB 460 L849h 1995]
RJ53.P5L66 1995
615.8′2′083—dc20
DNLM/DLC
for Library of Congress

94-38122
CIP

95 96 97 98 99
1 2 3 4 5 6 7 8 9 10

To our parents

Cecilia and Stanley Long

V. Lea Cody and J. Sidney Lea

Preface

Handbook of Pediatric Physical Therapy is a succinct yet comprehensive reference on the specialty area of pediatric physical therapy. The book covers the breadth of pediatric physical therapy in one accessible source. It provides all of the essential information needed by the student physical therapist, the generalist, and the novice pediatric physical therapist to assess or evaluate a child, design and implement a treatment plan, and determine when assistance from a more experienced pediatric physical therapist or other team member is needed.

In the face of an ever-changing health care delivery system, more and more therapists will be expected to initiate assessment and/or treatment for patients with whom they have had limited experience. Because time may be very limited, it is critical that therapists have necessary information in a convenient format to initiate an intervention plan. We have all experienced the trepidation of receiving a referral for a patient with a diagnosis we had not previously encountered, and we may have hastily tried to gather information by reviewing or scanning textbooks. Many times the research, academic, and/or didactic nature of these books did not prove immediately relevant, and we were left to our own clinical experience and, sometimes, intuition. The *Handbook of Pediatric Physical Therapy* has been designed to eliminate the tedious search for information.

A compendium of information organized in an accessible manner, the *Handbook* does not replace textbooks; it will complement them. Most of the information is in an outline format that allows the busy therapist to access information quickly for immediate application to a particular patient.

The *Handbook* is divided into six major chapters. Chapter 1, Growth and Development, presents information on the stages of development and on conditions and/or factors that may affect development. An emphasis on genetic disorders reflects today's rapidly expanding knowledge of the human genome. It also discusses the course of development for specific conditions, such as prematurity.

Chapter 2, Measurement, provides a basic foundation on the theory of measurement and the interpretation of standardized tests. This chapter contains information on clinical assessment strategies, such as strength testing and fitness testing in children, in addition to a comprehensive listing of assessment instruments, their psychometric properties, and their source.

In Chapter 3, Pediatric Disorders, we chose to use the Nagi adaptation of the WHO International classification of Impairment, Disability and Handicap (ICIDH). Each disorder is organized according to pathology and/or etiology, impairments, functional limitations, and treatment strategies. Rather than describe specific types or treatment perspectives, we present broad goals and treatment frameworks that are suited for each condition. We hope this will facilitate creativity in the therapist's design of a treatment plan and not promote one type of therapy over another or treatment by protocol. If the individual needs of a child and family are of utmost concern, we feel the therapist, given a treatment structure, will select specific treatment strategies and techniques to best meet those needs.

Chapter 4, Adaptive Equipment, presents those pieces of equipment that are unique to pediatric physical therapy and the purpose of each. We have tried to avoid repeating information that is basic to all physical therapists; for example, measuring for crutches or a standard wheelchair. We chose instead to describe treatment equipment, orthoses, and mobility devices unique to the needs of children with disabilities. In the section on treatment equipment, we have described and given basic treatment goals associated with each piece of equipment, again to assist the therapist with treatment planning. The section describing equipment used to promote sensorimotor or sensory integrative functioning should be especially helpful as some of this equipment may be unfamiliar to the physical therapist.

Locomotion, Chapter 5, reviews developmental changes leading to bipedal gait—from neonatal ambulation patterns through mature locomotor behavior. Gait assessment methods are outlined including the advantages and limitations of each. Atypical locomotor patterns are described as well as variations in the development of ambulation skills related to culture, physical attributes, and environmental factors.

Finally, Chapter 6, Administrative Issues, outlines the philosophical, legislative, and regulatory underpinnings of pediatric physical therapy. Administrative issues of hospital-based practice are covered briefly, as much of this information would be unique to the practice setting within a specific hospital. Additionally, the rapid changes in insurance coverage would make much of this information outdated before publication; however, basic information on coding is given. We have presented legal mandates that provide direction for practice and the evolution from practitioner-directed to family-guided practice. Differences between school-based therapy and early intervention are discussed as well as team structures, and the formats and benefits of each.

A Glossary, Resources, and Sources are also provided. The Glossary emphasizes terms that are unique to pediatric physical therapy. The Resources list a compilation of national associations and groups that the pediatric physical therapist may find helpful. The resources are divided into categories based on their primary purpose or focus such as advocacy, professional organizations, and clearinghouses. The Sources, organized by chapter, will provide direction for those seeking more detailed information.

Our goal is to facilitate, for the physical therapist and others in related fields, access to clinically relevant information in a practical format. We hope the *Handbook* will be a useful and handy resource for the reader. We welcome reader comments as we all continually strive to provide our young patients with the best possible care.

We would like to acknowledge our contributors, Kathy Harp, Andrea Santman Wiener, and Britta Battaile; and we thank the Book Division of Williams & Wilkins, particularly John Butler, for being enthusiastic about the concept right from the start, and Linda Napora, who advised, cajoled, and sometimes coerced us into completing the manuscript. Finally, Toby Long would like to thank Carol Schunk, a dear friend and colleague, for suggesting the idea for this book so many years ago.

Toby M. Long
Holly Lea Cintas

Contributors

Britta Battaile, M.S., P.T., P.C.S.

One Step Ahead
Physical Therapy Services
Bethesda, Maryland

Kathleen A. Harp, M.H.S., P.T., P.C.S.

Pediatric Physical Therapy
Rockville, Maryland

Andrea Santman Wiener, M.H.S., P.T., P.C.S.

Building Blocks, Pediatric Rehabilitation Services
Washington, D.C.

Contents

1 / Growth and Development

Holly Lea Cintas

Under optimal circumstances, a child is conceived, experiences an uneventful gestation and birth, and, with nurturing, achieves the independence of adulthood as a healthy human being. Pediatric therapists are frequently challenged by children and their families whose problems represent variations from the usual flow of developmental events. Many sources are available which describe growth and development based on parameters applicable to nondisabled children. The intent of this chapter is to utilize typical growth and development as a foundation in order to focus on the outcomes that occur when development is disrupted.

PRENATAL EVENTS AND GENETIC DISORDERS

Prenatal development begins with the fusion of the male germ cell, the sperm, and the female germ cell, the ovum, to form a **zygote:** the **genetic prototype** from which all remaining cells develop.

Meiosis

1. Cell division occurring prior to fertilization
2. Unique to formation of germ cells
3. Provides for random combination of genetic materials from each parent by production of **haploid** germ cells, which contain half the number of chromosomes found in other body cells

Mitosis

1. Cell division supporting continued growth and development of the organism after fertilization
2. **Diploid,** or complete chromosome number, is achieved by the combination of one paternal **X** or **Y** chromosome with one maternal **X** chromosome to produce an **XX** female or **XY** male having **44** autosomes

Genetic Disorders (See Table 1.1)

1. Can occur in association with meiosis prior to fertilization or mitosis following fertilization
2. Most common cause of birth defects; responsible for one third of all birth defects and about 85% of those with identified causes

Table 1.1. Examples of Genetic Disorders

Chromosome Number Abnormalities	Chromosome Structure Abnormalities	Gene Mutations
Monosomy	**Mosaicism**	**Autosomal Dominant Inheritance**
Turner syndrome: 45 XO	Down syndrome	Achondroplasia
		Ectrodactyly or polydactyly
	Translocation	Osteogenesis imperfecta
Trisomy	Down syndrome	
47 XYY syndrome	Trisomy 9 mosaic syndrome	**Autosomal Recessive Inheritance**
47 XXY syndrome		Cystic fibrosis
Trisomy 21: Down syndrome	**Chromosomal deletions**	Childhood spinal muscular atrophy (SMA types I, II, III)
Trisomy 18: Edwards' syndrome	Cri du chat syndrome	
Trisomy 13		**X-Linked Inheritance**
		Recessive
Tetrasomies	**Microdeletions**	Hemophilia
48 XXYY	Prader-Willi syndrome	Duchenne's muscular dystrophy
48 XXXY		Fragile X syndrome
	Angelman syndrome	Lesch-Nyhan syndrome
Pentasomies		
49 XXXYY		**Dominant**
49 XXXXX		Rett syndrome

CHROMOSOME NUMBER ABNORMALITIES

Nondisjunction error in cell division during meiosis results in unequal distribution of chromosomal material.

1. Ova or sperm produced have more or fewer than 23 chromosomes
2. Combination with a germ cell that has a normal complement of chromosomes produces zygote with numerical chromosome abnormality

Monosomy: only one of chromosome pair present at specific site.

1. Can be result of union of a sperm or ovum that has only 22 chromosomes with a normal germ cell
2. 99% of infants do not survive
3. Most common cytogenetic abnormality in spontaneous abortions
4. **45 XO (Turner syndrome)**
   a. Incidence in newborn females is between 1 in 3000 to 1 in 10,000
   b. Characteristics may include: transient congenital lymphedema, small stature evident

at birth, web-like appearance of the lateral neck, gonadal underdevelopment, hearing impairment, bone trabecular abnormalities

c. Cognitive deficiency, if present, attributable to chromosome abnormality other than XO

Trisomy: 3 of a particular chromosome at a specific site.

1. Zygote with 47 chromosomes produced when a germ cell with 24 chromosomes fuses with one that has 23 chromosomes
2. Trisomies of sex chromosomes common, but often go undetected until adolescence or adulthood because specific characteristics not apparent in infants
3. **47 XYY syndrome**
   a. Characterized by tall stature, shoulder girdle weakness, and generalized dyscoordination, especially fine motor
   b. Explosive behavioral outbursts and antisocial behaviors
   c. Incidence of XYY syndrome in incarcerated adolescents 24 times greater than in population of nondisabled newborn males
4. **47 XXY (Klinefelter syndrome)**
   a. Present in 1 in 500 males
   b. Most common cause of infertility in adult males
   c. Characteristics include hypogonadism, long limbs, and slim stature
   d. Obesity problematic in adults who have not received testosterone replacement therapy prior to adolescence
5. **Autosomal trisomies**
   a. Associated with significant growth abnormalities and cognitive delay
   b. Several autosomal trisomies exist, only three (**21, 18,** and **13**) are characterized by significant postnatal survival
6. **Trisomy 21 (Down syndrome)**
   a. Described in detail in Chapter 3
   b. Most frequent chromosomal disorder which is associated with moderate to severe cognitive delay
   c. Increased paternal and maternal ages thought to be contributing factors
   d. Trisomy 21 associated with 90% of cases of Down syndrome; remaining cases due to translocation or mosaicism
7. **Trisomy 18 (Edwards' syndrome)**
   a. Second most frequent disorder following trisomy 21
   b. Severe cognitive delay
   c. 90% of infants have significant cardiovascular, skeletal, urogenital, and gastrointestinal anomalies and do not survive beyond 1 year of age
   d. Fluctuations between hypotonicity and hypertonicity with increasing age
8. **Trisomy 13 (D_1 trisomy syndrome)**
   a. Limited life span; fewer than 5% of children survive beyond 3 years of age

b. Severe central nervous system anomalies common, such as holoprosencephaly associated with anophthalmia or microphthalmia, cleft lip and palate
c. Polydactyly, finger flexion contractures and rocker bottom feet associated with trisomy 13 and trisomy 18

Tetrasomies (48XXYY, 48XXXY) and pentasomies (49XXXYY, 49XXXXX)

1. Characterized by decreased stature, hypogenitalism, moderate to severe cognitive delay, and hypotonia
2. Children with these disorders display many features characteristic of Down syndrome
3. Genetic testing necessary for differential diagnosis

CHROMOSOME STRUCTURE ABNORMALITIES

Mosaicism

1. Typically results from a **nondisjunction error** during **mitotic** cell division
2. As zygote cells increase in number to become an embryo, some body cells carry normal chromosomal complement while others have atypical genotype
3. Occurs in sex chromosomes as well as autosomes
4. Children with mosaicism associated with a specific genetic condition have less severe physical and cognitive manifestations than those who are nonmosaic

Translocation

1. Breakage and transfer of chromosomal material to unrelated, intact chromosome pairs
2. Source of disorder in 3–4% of children with Down syndrome; extra 21st chromosome is attached to an intact chromosome other than 21
3. Basis for other, very rare trisomic syndromes such as **trisomy 9 mosaic syndrome**
4. Translocation not always associated with abnormal development; balanced translocation carrier with translocation between chromosomes 14 and 21 may be phenotypically normal with no external manifestation of the translocation

Chromosomal Deletion

1. Typically induced by chromosome breakage such as translocation, but broken portion is lost rather than reattached
2. Chromosome breaks that produce translocations and deletions usually result from environmental influences such as drugs, radiation, viruses, or chemical teratogens, rather than inheritance
3. **Cri du Chat syndrome**
    a. Results from a terminal deletion of the short arm of chromosome 5
    b. Abnormal laryngeal development results in characteristic weak and high-pitched cry
    c. Cognitive deficit and microcephaly uniformly present

   d. Hypotonia, hypertelorism, and scoliosis frequently present
   e. Congenital heart abnormalities in 30% of infants
   f. Significantly higher level of intellectual performance associated with home rearing rather than institutionalization
4. **Microdeletions** can span several contiguous genes
   a. Identified by means of high-resolution chromosome banding techniques
   b. **Prader-Willi syndrome** and **Angelman syndrome** are **contiguous gene syndromes**
      - Each disorder is associated with a specific deletion of band q12 on chromosome 15
      - Whether the child will have Prader-Willi or Angelman syndrome depends on which parent contributes deleted chromosome 15
      - **Prader-Willi syndrome**
         - Father source of the deletion
         - Characteristics include mild cognitive delay, hypotonia during infancy, short stature, and hyperphagia, which can result in severe obesity
         - Prader-Willi-like syndrome has been described in males as a subtype of **Fragile X syndrome**
      - **Angelman (Happy Puppet syndrome)**
         - Deletion present in the mother
         - Associated with severe cognitive delay, microcephaly, seizures, ataxia contributing to a "puppet-like" gait, and frequent laughter

GENE MUTATIONS AND MODES OF INHERITANCE

Specific gene mutations are the basis for 7–8% of congenital anomalies.

1. Loss or change of function of a gene is permanent and inheritable once mutation has occurred
2. Congenital anomalies from gene mutations inherited according to Mendelian genetics; probabilities of their occurrence are predictable
3. Some gene mutations fatal; most have undesirable consequences
4. Mutations can occur randomly; environmental agents such as radiation and carcinogenic chemicals known to increase rate of occurrence

Autosomal Dominant Inheritance

1. Mutant gene contributed by one parent
2. Predicted risk of offspring inheriting the disorder is 50%; phenotypic expression may be well below 50%; wide variation in the manifestation of disorder due to single, rather than dual, parent contribution
3. If new (fresh) gene mutation occurred in single germ cell participating in fertilization, risk of another child with same syndrome negligible; increased parental age is a risk factor for new mutations

4. **Achondroplasia**
   a. Most frequent cause of short stature
   b. Disturbance of endochondral ossification at epiphyseal plate
   c. New mutations responsible for 80–90% of the incidence
   d. Older paternal age significant contributing factor to new mutations in achondroplasia and several other autosomal dominant malformation syndromes
   e. Characteristics may include bilateral shortness of humerus and femur, and macrocephaly associated with hydrocephalus at birth
   f. 46% of children with achondroplasia have spinal complications: kyphosis, stenosis of the spinal canal, or disc lesions
5. **Ectrodactyly:** cleft hand or cleft foot in which two or more digits are fused, creating a central opening
6. **Polydactyly**
   a. Extra digits present on the hand or foot
   b. Most limb defects due to genetic factors, although **maternal thalidomide** ingestion linked to limb anomalies such as **phocomelia**
7. **Osteogenesis Imperfecta**
   a. Error in collagen development associated with multiple fractures
   b. **Four types:** three, **I, II,** and **IV,** are **autosomal dominant** and result from spontaneous mutation; minimal likelihood of recurrence. **Type III** is **autosomal recessive** and associated with abnormally short, angled, and bowed limbs, scoliosis after puberty, and normal sclerae
   c. **Type IV** is mild form associated with osteoporosis, normal sclerae, and limited incidence and severity of fractures
   d. **Type II** is congenitally lethal; infants are stillborn or typically die within perinatal period; blue sclerae are diagnostic for types I and II
   e. Infants with **type I** have good prognosis for survival and are excellent candidates for active physical therapy
      - Long leg bones most frequent fracture sites
      - Periods of highest fracture incidence are 2–3 years and 10–15 years
      - Fractures decrease following adolescence, although this can be negatively affected by pregnancy, lactation, or periods of inactivity

Autosomal Recessive Inheritance

1. Both parents transmit gene mutation
2. Predicted risk of offspring having the disorder is 25% if parents are heterozygous (unaffected carriers)
3. If both parents are homozygous and have same autosomal recessive disorder, potential for transmission to offspring is high and further increased by consanguinity
4. **Cystic fibrosis** is an autosomal recessive disorder described in Chapter 3
5. **Childhood spinal muscular atrophy (SMA)**

   a. Anterior horn cell degeneration and flaccid paralysis
   b. Muscle biopsy and EMG confirm diagnosis
   c. Intelligence, social development, sensation, and sphincter function unaffected
   d. **Three types:** diagnosis prior to 1 year of age corresponds to **SMA 1,** 1–4 years to **SMA 2,** and 5–15 years to **SMA 3**
   e. Symptoms of **infantile** form, **SMA 1 (Werdnig- Hoffman disease),** may include decreased fetal movements in third trimester, postnatal poor head control, hypotonia, and widely abducted extremities
      - Proximal, symmetrical weakness often identified first followed by respiratory and feeding difficulties
      - Survival beyond 3 years of age rare
   f. **Childhood** form, **SMA 2** (chronic Werdnig-Hoffman disease), has similar patterns of weakness, but slower progression and more optimistic prognosis
      - May be evident after 3–6 months of age as motor milestone delay becomes apparent
      - Feeding rarely problematic
      - Functional ambulation with assistive devices may be possible
   g. **Juvenile** form, **SMA 3 (Kugelberg-Welander Disease),** characterized by mild, progressive weakness in proximal muscles
      - Differential diagnosis is necessary to rule out Muscular Dystrophy
      - Contractures and spinal asymmetry rarely problematic

X-linked Inheritance

1. Transmitted on the X-chromosome
2. Males primarily affected; females minimally affected or may be unaffected carriers
3. Males born to a carrier mother have a 50% chance of inheriting X-linked disorder; daughters have a 50% chance of becoming carriers
4. Affected daughter has inherited a mutant allele from both parents, or her normal X chromosome has been inactivated
5. **X-linked dominant** disorders extremely rare and usually lethal in males; among more than 14,000 X-linked congenital disorders identified, fewer than 10 are attributed to X-linked dominance
6. **Rett syndrome**
   a. Hypothesized to be X-linked dominant because present in females only; lethal in males before birth
   b. First 6 months' normal development followed by gradual loss of cognitive, communication, and motor skills, deceleration of head growth, onset of hypotonia, and ataxia
   c. Often diagnosed initially as autism due to trunk rocking, absence of eye contact, and language disorder
   d. Unique characteristics are stereotyped, repetitive hand wringing, tapping, or mouthing
7. **Hemophilia** and **Duchenne's muscular dystrophy** are **X-linked recessive** disorders discussed in Chapter 3

8. **Fragile X syndrome**
   a. X-linked recessive disorder characterized by normal life span
   b. Most common cause of mental retardation in males after Down syndrome
   c. Older paternal age associated with carrier status in females
   d. Characteristics may include increased head circumference, prominent forehead, generalized hypotonia, torticollis, and scoliosis
9. **Lesch-Nyhan syndrome**
   a. X-linked recessive disorder with excessive production of uric acid and deleterious effects on the brain and liver
   b. Onset of spasticity at 6–8 months of age, subsequent choreoathetosis, growth deficiency, and autism
   c. Metabolic markers for this disorder detectable by amniocentesis
   d. Distinguished by tendency of children to self-mutilate; may begin with lip biting at 1–2 years of age and progress to other body parts such as the fingers

ENVIRONMENTAL INFLUENCES ON PRENATAL DEVELOPMENT

Environmental Agents

Environmental agents such as radiation, heavy metals, infectious or chemical teratogens contribute to chromosome abnormalities, especially deletion and translocation, and increase the rate of gene mutations. Multifactorial inheritance occurs when genetic and environmental factors work synergistically to produce anomalies. Environmental factors acting independently are responsible for 7–10% of congenital malformations. Anomalies due to maternal drug or alcohol ingestion or infection may appear to be genetic conditions when 2 or more children of typical parents have the same disorder; differentiation of inherited disorders from those resulting from an environmental agent is critical for family counseling and prevention of birth defects.

Impact of Timing

The means by which environmental teratogens act on developing tissue is undocumented in most cases, but the timing of an environmental insult correlates with the outcome.

1. **First 2 weeks** following fertilization: **embryonic death** is typical outcome of teratogenic activity
2. **Weeks 3–8**
   a. Most susceptible interval for production of multisystem congenital anomalies
   b. Rapid cell division and tissue differentiation leading to organ development are the basis for teratogenic sensitivity
   c. Maternal **rubella** infection during this period carries a 50% risk of embryonic infection
      - Anomalies reflect systems undergoing rapid differentiation: eye, ear, heart, blood vessels, and brain

   - Rubella virus can remain in the infant's tissues and cause ongoing complications following birth

   d. **Critical periods** for specific structures may extend beyond this interval. Critical period for brain development is 3–16 weeks' gestational age, but brain continues to develop rapidly for 2 years following birth. Extended period for brain development makes CNS sensitive to effects of maternal alcohol ingestion throughout pregnancy, contributing to risk of **Fetal Alcohol syndrome (FAS)**

3. **Weeks 9–38**
   a. Most tissues already differentiated and less sensitive to teratogenic influences; brain is an exception
      - Chronic cognitive deficit accompanied by microcephaly is frequent response to infections or other environmental insults during this interval
      - **Toxoplasmosis**
        - Maternal infection can result from contact with uncooked meat or eggs, unpasteurized milk, soil, or cat feces containing toxoplasma cysts
        - Transplacental fetal infection associated with hydrocephalus, microcephaly, and cerebral palsy
      - **Cytomegalovirus (CMV), herpes simplex virus (HSV), varicella (chickenpox), human immunodeficiency virus (HIV), and syphilis**
        - All may result in microcephaly and/or cognitive delay
        - Infant may not be infected until vaginal delivery
      - Pregnant woman may be unaware of infected status with respect to toxoplasmosis, CMV, or HIV
      - Treatment of the mother with **syphilis** before the 16th week of pregnancy can prevent transplacental fetal infection

   b. **Rubella** infection occurring after 1st trimester carries low risk of anomalies; no documented anomalies associated with rubella infection after the 5th gestational month, although chronic visual, auditory, or central nervous system dysfunction may still occur

   c. Impact of **thalidomide** ingestion also highly time-dependent
      - Complete absence of an arm or leg (amelia) associated with 24–36 days' gestational age
      - Mild to moderate defects are associated with later ingestion during 1st trimester
      - No available clinical evidence links thalidomide ingestion with embryonic maldevelopment after first trimester

MATERNAL SUBSTANCE ABUSE (SEE TABLE 1.2)

Alcohol Ingestion and Fetal Alcohol Syndrome (FAS)

1. Described in the 1960s, but impact of maternal alcohol ingestion on fetal development and frequency of occurrence not recognized until the 1990s

Table 1.2. Effects of Maternal Substance Use

Substance	Pregnancy Complications	Neonatal Complications	Childhood Health and Development
Cigarettes	Miscarriage Prematurity, IUGR Pre-eclampsia Placental abruption Placenta previa	Low birth weight Increased risk of SIDS Increased neonatal mortality	Slow growth Learning disabilities Behavioral problems Respiratory disease during first 5 years
Alcohol	Miscarriage Poor weight gain Anemia Hepatitis	Withdrawal Low birth weight Restlessness Poor sucking	Fetal alcohol effect or Fetal alcohol syndrome: Flattened nasal bridge & philtrum Epicantal folds Microcephaly Learning disorders Hyperactivity Joint, cardiac anomalies Hearing, visual deficits
Opiates (methadone, heroin)	Prematurity Toxemia	Withdrawal High-pitched cry Irritability, seizures Fever, seizures Sleep disturbance, diarrhea Tremulousness Poor feeding, vomiting Increased risk of SIDS	Developmental delay Learning disabilities Hyperactivity Hearing deficit Visual impairment

Table 1.2. continued

Substance	Pregnancy Complications	Neonatal Complications	Childhood Health and Development
Cocaine	Prematurity Hypertension Tachycardia Placental abruption Precipitous delivery Poor weight gain Slow intrauterine growth	Withdrawal, irritability Stroke Disturbed sleep Restlessness Hyperreflexia Poor feeding Microcephaly	Cognitive retardation Learning disabilities Behavior problems CNS deficits Dyscoordination

2. Present in all socioeconomic groups
3. Considered by some to be the foremost documented cause of mental retardation in the western world
4. Most effective intervention is prospective parent education
5. Not all children exposed in utero display **alcohol-related birth defects (ARBD)** or more subtle deficits characteristic of **fetal alcohol effect (FAE)**
   a. Intrauterine growth retardation and impaired postnatal growth
   b. Central nervous system maldevelopment often with microcephaly
   c. Facial and joint dysmorphology
   d. Cardiac, renal, genital, and immunological anomalies
6. Difficult to determine amount sufficient to induce teratogenic effects since **no general agreement** on **minimum safe dose**
   a. Growth retardation associated with as few as two drinks per day
   b. Amount of alcohol ingested by the mother is less important than the peak blood alcohol levels attained in the fetus
      - Fetal alcohol elimination, passively dependent on the placenta, occurs at a slower rate than maternal elimination
      - Fetus at risk for exposure to much higher doses of alcohol for longer periods than the mother
   c. High-volume binge drinking especially risky
7. Children with FAS have multiple, although sometimes subtle, developmental problems, and considerable individual variation
   a. Hypotonia, early feeding difficulties, and delayed motor milestones typical in infants
   b. Gross motor delays persist as subtle balance and coordination problems in older children
   c. Fine motor limitations more apparent with age and increasing educational expectations

   d. Above average incidence of scoliosis, rib cage anomalies, congenital hip dislocation, clubfoot, and other joint abnormalities
   e. Mild to moderate cognitive impairment may be complicated by presence of attention deficit hyperactivity disorder (ADHD) or autism

Maternal Drug Use

1. Difficult to determine effects of specific drugs on the fetus because maternal substance abuse often includes multiple drugs
   a. Further confounded by prematurity, adverse environmental factors, and genetic effects
   b. Research studies report a range of outcomes from no specific developmental sequelae to CNS impairment; animal studies have shown a wide continuum of effects from prenatal death to subtle behavioral variations
2. Neonatal behaviors may be highly aberrant but of short duration; abnormal behaviors include tremulousness, sleep disorders, poor state control, hyperirritability, and ineffectual sucking
3. Once infants have stabilized, developmental scores typically within normal limits, but significantly lower than matched groups with no history of maternal drug abuse
4. Negative impact on play behavior in toddlers has been reported, manifested as excessive throwing and dropping of toys, but interplay of many factors precludes determination of specific causality

MULTIPLE BIRTHS AND BIRTH DEFECTS

Birth defects are the result of chance, for example, fresh mutation, genetic effects, environmental effects, or an interaction of factors; the impact of these factors in multiple births depends on:

1. Whether infants are monozygotic or multizygotic
2. Their genders
3. Availability of intrauterine space
4. Placental blood supply

There has been a **26% increase** in multiple births since 1970.

1. Twin births now account for 1 in 43 of all births
2. Incidence of triplet births has tripled
3. Higher frequency of multiple births due to reproductive technology has increased potential for negative outcomes; incidence of cerebal palsy at least 6 times higher in twins than in single births
4. Trend toward delaying childbirth also contributes to increased incidence of birth defects
   a. Multiple births occur with greater frequency in older women

   b. Advanced parental age also associated with increased frequency of birth defects unrelated to multiple births

Monozygotic twins: Union of a single ovum with a single sperm

1. Presumed to be identical, but microscopic photon exposures, physical, or mechanical forces can negatively affect one twin to produce deformations such as club foot or hip dysplasia
2. Differential blood flow to each twin due to placental vessel anastomoses can create wide variation in intrauterine growth
3. Malformation rate in monozygotic twins 2–3 times higher than in dizygotic twins or singleton births

Dizygotic twins: fertilizations of two ova by two different sperm

1. No more similar than sisters and brothers born separately
2. Represent about ⅔ of all twins
3. Familial tendency for dizygotic twinning
4. Environmental risk factors common to monozygotic as well as dizygotic twins: in utero crowding, maternal infections, advanced parental age, trauma, birth order, radiation, and substance abuse

Conjoined (Siamese) twins: incompletely separated at embryonic disk stage during second and third week of gestation

1. Occurs about once in every 40 monozygotic twin pregnancies
2. Wide spectrum of linkages: superficial juncture of skin only to portion of one **parasitic twin** adherent to the body of the other

Twin death during the prenatal period not uncommon

1. Ultrasound examinations have identified early loss and reabsorption of one fetus with no deleterious effects on the surviving fetus
2. Can confound the results of prenatal tissue sampling such as **chorionic villus sampling (CVS)**
3. Rarely, emboli or thromboplastin entering the circulation of the surviving twin results in intravascular coagulation and tissue destruction leading to limb amputation or other sequelae

Multiple births: may be monozygotic, multizygotic, or any mixture of these types occurring in same gestational interval

1. Potential for birth defects related to fetal crowding increases proportionally to the number of fetuses; highest incidence of structural defects in monozygotic births
2. Some specific defects associated with multiplicity
   a. Higher than average incidence of the **VATER** association (vertebral anomalies, ventricular septal defect, tracheoesophageal fistula, and radial dysplasia)

b. Sacrococcygeal teratoma
c. Holoprosencephaly and anencephaly

DYSMORPHOLOGY

Malformations or malformation sequences: result of primary tissue defects originating **within** embryo or fetus.

1. Identified genetic disorders account for only about ⅓ of congenital malformations; remaining presumed multifactorial
2. **Sequence** is cascade of subsequent anomalies that can follow a single, primary malformation
3. **Syndrome** denotes multiple independent anomalies that develop from one primary cause
4. **Down syndrome** and **Osteogenesis Imperfecta** are examples of malformation syndromes

Disruptions by External Agents

1. Cause breakdown of fetal tissues developing normally up to that point
2. Infectious, vascular, or mechanical
3. **Fetal rubella syndrome** and **fetal alcohol syndrome** are examples of disruptions created by maternal infection or an environmental agent
4. Mechanical compression of the embryo secondary to premature amnion rupture can result in deformities such as amputation, syndactyly, or scoliosis

Deformations or deformation sequences: result of atypical mechanical forces altering normal development.

1. Typically due to extrinsic forces such as intrauterine position or constraint of an otherwise normal fetus
2. Occasionally can be a secondary outcome of an intrinsic factor within the fetus, such as a malformation
3. In general, deformations are far less serious than malformations; most have optimistic prognoses. Exception is most severe form of fetal constraint called **oligohydramnios sequence.**
   - Amniotic fluid insufficiency late in gestation due to chronic leakage or faulty fetal urine production
   - Diminished fetal growth, respiratory suppression, and multiple joint contractures

GROWTH: INFLUENCES AND PROGRESSION

Growth regulation is highly complex, dependent upon the interaction of nutritive, genetic, hormonal, mechanical, and environmental factors. Charts describing norms for growth parameters such as height, weight, head size, and progress of ossification (bone age) are available in many sources (see Sources and Recommended Readings).

Fetal growth depends on the physical size of the mother's uterus under normal conditions.

1. Insufficient space due to multiple fetuses or uterine abnormality may create joint deformations, especially clubfoot and hip dislocation
2. Growth deficiency due to constraint in late gestation usually compensated by catch-up growth following birth
3. First child is pacesetter whose role is to stretch the mother's uterus; typically weighs 200–300 g less than siblings
4. **Intrauterine growth retardation (IUGR)** may result from maternal malnutrition, illness, placental insufficiency, or exposure to toxic agents such as alcohol, heavy metals, or drugs
5. Infants of mothers with **insulin** dependent diabetes are frequently large for gestational age
6. Neonatal size typically unaffected by hypothyroidism or growth hormone insufficiency, but thyroid hormone essential for fetal skeletal maturation

Average birth weight is between 5.5 (2500 g) and 9 lb.

1. **AGA** (appropriate /average for gestational age): birth weight between 10th and 90th percentiles for infant's gestational age
2. **LGA** (large for gestational age): birth weight > 90th percentile
3. **SGA** (small for gestational age): birth weight < 10th percentile
4. **LBW** (low birth weight): < 2500 g
   a. Full-term infant weighing < 5.5 lb considered SGA and LBW
   b. Preterm infant weighing < 5.5 lb considered LBW but not necessarily SGA
5. **VLBW** (very low birth weight): < 1500 g
6. **ELBW** (extremely low birth weight): <1000 g
7. **Micropreemie:** <750 g

Parents' combined height (mid-parental height) is major determinant of the child's ultimate stature (see Tables 1.3 and 1.4).

1. Very premature infant can achieve height of 6 or 7 ft
2. Multiple factors can interfere with the individual's ability to achieve genetically programmed adult stature (see Tables 1.3–1.5)
3. **Nutrition** critical factor
   a. Growth deficiency resulting from malnutrition can be overcome to some extent by catch-up growth
   b. Growth deficits due to malnutrition after the end of the 4th year can be fully compensated by catch-up growth
   c. Insufficient nutrition during first 4 years indelibly reduces ultimate stature; cannot be reversed by optimal conditions after 4 years of age

Growth **appears to be but is not a continuous process** with specific accelerations in velocity, for example, adolescent growth spurt.

1. Growth in length during the first 21 months of age occurs in discontinuous, aperiodic bursts ranging from 0.5–2.5 cm
2. No measurable growth may occur for as long as 63 days
3. Growth during infancy actually occurs less than 10% of the time in transient bursts
4. Short-term inhibitors such as illness are easily remediated by catch-up growth, but not if condition is severe or chronic

Hormones are critical influences on growth.

1. Appropriate amounts of **growth hormone (GH), thyroxin,** and **insulin** essential throughout development to achieve adequate stature
2. **Gonadal sex hormones** coordinate with GH to provide the adolescent growth spurt
   a. These are under hypothalamic-pituitary control, as are GH and thyroxin; short stature may result from pituitary tumors
   b. Adrenal androgens do not appear to have major impact on growth
3. **Somatomedin-C (Sm-C),** produced by the liver, directly stimulates skeletal growth prenatally and postnatally
   a. Similar or possibly identical to insulin-like growth factor **(IGF-I)**
   b. May be common denominator coordinating the effects of other growth factors
      - Production increased by GH and insulin and decreased by malnutrition, estrogen treatment, and possibly corticosteroids
      - Rapid growth associated with increased GH production and low serum levels of Sm-C during infancy, perhaps indicative of negative feedback relationship between the two hormones
      - Late adolescence characterized by relatively high concentrations of serum Sm-C during growth rate deceleration

Failure to Thrive (FTT) is a growth deficiency occurring during infancy and early childhood.

1. Attributable to psychosocial and/or biological factors
2. Should be considered in nonambulatory children less than 2 years of age having low weight for length and no evidence of organic disease
3. Length, weight, and height usually below the 3rd percentile for age
4. Environmental contributors include inadequate nutrition, inconsistent parenting, and environmental neglect
5. Evidence of organic disease is present in fewer than 50% of children typically diagnosed with FTT
   a. Organic and environmental factors may interact
   b. Gastrointestinal or neurological disorders, or both, are primary organic sources of FTT

Table 1.3. Growth Disorders Associated with Excessive Height

Type	Source of Disorder	Significant Signs	Other
Beckwith-Wiedemann syndrome	Cause unknown; families in which more than 1 sibling affected have been reported	Excessive growth rate in infancy decelerates later; macrosomia; macroglossia	High incidence of prematurity; hemihypertrophy may be present on one side of body
Fragile X syndrome	X-linked inheritance, fragile site is at Xq27	Growth rate in infancy may resemble cerebral gigantism	Hypotonia, cognitive delay, delayed motor milestones
Homocystinuria syndrome	Autosomal recessive enzyme deficiency resulting in skeletal and visual dysplasias	Failure to thrive with growth deficiency may occur, but normal to tall stature common; lens subluxation by age 10	Seizures, arachnodactyly, multiple joint malalignment; osteoporosis; dietary treatment may be effective
Marfan's syndrome	Autosomal dominant; connective tissue disorder of undetermined origin	Tall stature associated with little subcutaneous fat, joint laxity with high incidence of scoliosis and kyphosis	Arachnodactyly; normal intelligence; cardiovascular defects such as aortic aneurysm or mitral prolapse may lead to sudden death
Neurofibromatosis	Autosomal dominant with wide variance of expression; multiple system abnormalities	Excessive height may be present in addition to subcutaneous, central nervous system and skeletal tumors	Cognitive deficiency in very few children; seizures; syndactyly; scoliosis; hypoplastic bowing lower legs

Table 1.3. continued

Type	Source of Disorder	Significant Signs	Other
Normal Variance	No evident abnormality; tall parents; may have increased serum levels of somadomedin-C or insulin-like growth factor	Height above 95th percentile; if bone age is advanced, growth potential is limited and ultimate height may be within acceptable range	Estrogen therapy may be attempted in females to hasten epiphyseal fusion, but side effects associated with significant risk
Pituitary Gigantism	Pituitary tumor; fasting levels of growth hormone elevated	Excessive growth is proportional throughout body; no distinguishing facial features	Acromegaly occurs if tumor becomes active after epiphyseal fusion; limited success with surgery, radiation
Sotos syndrome (cerebral gigantism)	Cause unknown; may be autosomal dominant; possible congenital hypothalamic abnormality	Large at birth; rapid growth continues during childhood but final height may be within normal limits	Hands, feet, and skull unusually large; dilated cerebral ventricles; cognitive retardation
Weaver syndrome	Cause unknown; may be autosomal dominant or X-linked recessive	Accelerated prenatal growth and advanced skeletal maturation during infancy	Progressive spasticity; foot deformities and flexion contractures typical

Table 1.4. Growth Disorders Associated with Short Stature

Type	Source of Disorder	Significant Signs	Other
Achondroplasia	Autosomal dominant; most common chondrodysplasia; new mutations responsible for 90% of occurrences; paternal age a factor	Insufficient epiphyseal growth; short extremities, head large, with frontal bossing; hydrocephalus and cord compression may occur due to narrow foramen magnum	Early sitting, standing, and walking discouraged because of weight of large head and proportionately short extremities to minimize lumbar lordosis and bowing
Central nervous system disorders, especially with cognitive delay	Multiple causes; injury to hypothalamus may affect hypothalamic-pituitary regulation of growth	Global motor and cognitive delay; often accompanied by oral-motor dyscoordination and gastroesophageal reflux	Growth failure may be due to one or several nutritional, physiological, anatomical, or environmental factors
Chronic pulmonary disease	Malnutrition major factor; lung disease more significant than malabsorption in cystic fibrosis	Minimal subcutaneous fat; distal digital clubbing with advanced lung disease	Steroidal treatment for asthma may further retard growth
Congenital heart disease	Insufficient tissue nutrition may result from poor cardiovascular dynamics	Growth poorest in children with cyanotic heart disease, but compensatory growth often follows surgical correction	Serum levels of growth hormone same as in nondisabled children

Table 1.4. continued

Type	Source of Disorder	Significant Signs	Other
De Lange syndrome (Cornelia de Lange syndrome)	Unknown cause; autosomal dominance suggested, based on two affected siblings born to mildly involved parent	Prenatal onset, short stature, delayed osseous maturation, small limbs, thin downturned upper lip characteristic	Motor delay, hypertonia in infancy, multiple joint deformations, cognitive delay, feeding difficulties, seizures
Fetal alcohol syndrome (FAS)	Maternal alcohol ingestion during pregnancy; abstinence most effective intervention	Prenatal and postnatal growth deficiency; multiple facial abnormalities, microcephaly	Moderate to severe cognitive impairment and generalized developmental delay; hyperactivity
Growth hormone insufficiency	May be familial: autosomal recessive or dominant, X-linked recessive; may be due to pituitary tumor, especially craniopharyngioma	High incidence of perinatal problems: excessive vaginal bleeding during gestation, breech delivery, perinatal asphyxia	High pitched voice, immature facies, excessive breast and abdominal fat; treatment with synthetically produced growth hormone before epiphyseal fusion
Heavy metal insufficiency or abundance	Nutritional zinc insufficiency or high serum concentrations of lead	Anorexia and poor growth with insufficient zinc	Nervous system dysfunction and general malaise with lead toxicity

Table 1.4. continued

Type	Source of Disorder	Significant Signs	Other
Hypochondroplasia	Autosomal dominant, but majority of cases result from new mutations when parents are unaffected	Marked shortening of long bones, normal craniofacial appearance; bowing of legs, milder than achondroplasia	Rare occurrence compared with achondrodysplasia, but incidence of cognitive deficit much higher than achondroplasia
Malabsorption and inflammatory bowel syndromes: celiac disease, Crohn's disease	Nutritional deficiency due to malabsorption; secondary hypopituitarism may co-exist	Proportionally small stature which can be compensated if intervention occurs before puberty	Growth may be enhanced by successful steroidal therapy or surgical intervention
Metaphyseal Chondroplasia, McKusick type (Cartilage-hair Hypoplasia)	Autosomal recessive; irregular scalloped metaphyses; gastrointestinal malabsorption often early problem which resolves with time	Short stature due to short extremities; fine, sparse hair; joint hypermobility, although elbow flexion contractures common	Susceptibility to chicken pox infection may be fatal due to a cellular immune deficit
Metaphyseal Dysostosis	Autosomal dominant; insufficient mineralization of primary calcification areas in the metaphyses	Severe short stature, postnatal onset, limited if any craniofacial involvement; flexion deformities of joints	Waddling gait, deafness may be present

Table 1.4. continued

Type	Source of Disorder	Significant Signs	Other
Primordial or familial short stature	No obvious abnormality; may have short parents; typically small for gestational age	Small size is proportional, except for head size which correlates with chronological age; bone age proportional to chronological age rather than height	Normal intelligence, sexual maturation, endocrine function; no evidence of abnormality except short stature which may be less than 4 feet
Renal disease, especially congenital urinary tract deficits or renal tubular acidosis	Acidosis, chronic malnutrition, renal rickets	Typically no external signs of primary disorder, only growth retardation; exception is high association of external ear malformation with congenital urinary tract defects	
Rickets	Vitamin D deficiency or X-linked Vitamin D-Resistant rickets (X-linked dominant) or Pseudo-vitamin D Deficiency Rickets (autosomal recessive)	Growth deficiency secondary to hypophosphatemia, hypocalcemia, perhaps insufficient absorption of calcium, phosphorus through intestinal tract	Bowing of legs, coxa vara, hypotonia, fractures; vitamin deficiency rickets and pseudo-vitamin deficiency rickets respond to high doses of vitamin D

Table 1.4. continued

Type	Source of Disorder	Significant Signs	Other
Seckel syndrome	Autosomal recessive inheritance	Prenatal onset of severe growth deficiency, associated with microcephaly, micrognathia, prominent nose	Moderate to severe cognitive deficit, although early motor progress may be near normal; at risk for joint deformations
Silver-Russell syndrome (Silver syndrome)	Unknown cause; may be tentative diagnosis for any small for gestational age infant	Prenatal onset of small stature; limb asymmetry common, triangular face, 5th finger incurvation	Motor delay common, although intelligence usually normal; gradual improvement in growth approaching adulthood
Turner syndrome (XO syndrome)	45, XO genetic complement or mosaic pattern such as XX/XO; edematous hands or feet may be a marker in the neonate	Short stature, wide neck, broad trunk, lack of breast development; dysplastic ovaries, cardiovascular defects, hearing impairment	Osteoporosis often present related to estrogen deficiency; deficit in spatial ability or visual memory may mask normal intelligence

Table 1.5. Growth Disorders Associated with Hemihypertrophy or Extremity Asymmetry

Type	Source of Disorder	Significant Signs	Other
Beckwith-Wiedemann syndrome	Cause unknown; families in which more than one sibling affected have been reported	Infantile gigantism; growth rate decreases over time	Hemihypertrophy: one half of body may be significantly larger than the other
CHILD syndrome (Congenital hemidysplasia with ichthyosiform erythroderma and limb defects)	Unknown cause	Unilateral growth deficiency of extremities varies from absence to hypoplasia of metacarpals, metatarsals, phalanges	Can include unilateral hypoplasia of any skeletal bones, cardiac septal defects, erythema, and scaling skin
Klippel-Trenaunay-Weber syndrome	Unknown cause; occurs sporadically, often in conjunction with hemangioma and/or atriovenous fistula	Congenital or early childhood hypertrophy of usually one limb, but can exceed one	Joint discomfort, leg swelling common; epiphyseal fusion may be utilized to minmize asymmetry; amputation rare
Leg length discrepancy	Paralysis, epiphyseal fracture, atriovenous malformation, fused joint	Asymmetrical bone growth due to interference with or acceleration of growth	High doses of ultrasound can interfere with epiphyseal development
Osteochondromatosis syndrome	Unknown cause; typically sporadic but has been reported to occur in more than one family member	Asymmetrical bone growth first noted at age 1–4 years; minimal progression after adolescence	Increased risk of fractures; reactivation of growth in adulthood should be evaluated for chondrosarcoma

Table 1.5. continued

Type	Source of Disorder	Significant Signs	Other
Proteus syndrome	Unknown cause; all reported cases have been sporadic	Asymmetric overgrowth of any external structure; increased stature, macrocephaly	Hemihypertrophy associated with bony prominences, angulation defects in knees, scoliosis, soft tissue tumors
Russell-Silver syndrome (Silver syndrome)	Unknown cause	Short stature a consistent feature; short and/or incurved 5th finger	Limb asymmetry common

- CNS impairment may create a cycle of low responsiveness, poor feeding patterns, malnutrition, and infection leading to further neurological impairment and FTT
- Anatomical, physiological, and infectious gastrointestinal disorders may contribute to a similar downward spiral
- Gastroesophageal reflux **(GER)** results in decreased nutritional intake due to anorexia, vomiting, or frequent respiratory tract infections

6. Hypothyroidism, hypopituitarism, severe cardiovascular or renal disease, and fetal alcohol syndrome may contribute to growth failure
7. Growth deficiency related to cystic fibrosis well known; elevated sweat electrolytes may also be present in children with nonorganic failure to thrive
8. Severe FTT associated with acquired immune deficiency syndrome

BIOMECHANICAL ASPECTS OF GROWTH

Mechanical forces, mediated by genetic and chemical factors, influence the child's growth from the earliest weeks of development.

1. Rate, shape, and volume of growth of one tissue source determine magnitude and direction of forces placed on neighboring tissues
2. **Plasticity** of adjacent tissues leads to complex series of negotiations to constrain or allow growth
   a. Extends throughout the growth period to meet anatomical and physiological deadlines in a flexible manner
   b. Places growing child at risk if mechanical forces are abnormal
   c. Basis for efficacy of therapeutic interventions to redirect atypical growth with taping, casting, orthotics, or surgery
3. **Movement** an essential factor to complete joint development during second and third prenatal months
   a. Joint development begins with dissolution of mesenchymal tissue to create cavities which eventually become fluid filled
   b. If stresses provided by prenatal movement are diminished or absent, joint dysplasias can lead to contracture or dislocation
      - **Fetal akinesia sequence** results in **multiple congenital contractures (arthrogryposis)**
      - Infants with paralytic **spina bifida** demonstrate same prenatal phenomenon, but to a lesser extent
   c. Diminished stress provided by muscle pull over several years has significant impact on leg length and ultimate height of children with lower extremity paralysis
4. **Muscle cells** align developmentally according to the direction of pull placed upon them
   a. Size and fiber type depend upon heredity, age, demand placed on them, gender, and presence of an intact electroneuromuscular apparatus to drive them
   b. Muscles appear much more compliant than bone to tensile stresses, i.e., they re-

spond to stretch by lengthening; tension forces which intact muscles place on bone are essential to bone development and joint alignment

5. **Bone** appears noncompliant compared to muscle, but is actually highly dynamic
   a. Grows in length and by apposition; interior reabsorption occurs simultaneously in response to hereditary, mechanical, nutritive, and hormonal influences
   b. **Wolff's law** describes association between bone structure and mechanical demands placed on it
      - Moderately high, consistent mechanical stresses increase bone density via deposition of periosteal and subperiosteal bone
      - Exceedingly high or low mechanical forces on bone result in resorption and decreased bone density
   c. Same quality which underlies transition from mesenchymal membrane (**intramembranous ossification**) or cartilage (**endochondral ossification**) to bone allows it to be modeled by **tension, compression,** and **torsional forces,** especially those exerted by muscles
      - **Leg length discrepancy** secondary to unilateral paralysis demonstrates influence of muscle pull on bone
      - Weightbearing known to have stimulatory effect on fracture healing, but muscle pull more significant to maintain density
      - Historical examples of bone modeling include skull elongation and foot molding through wrapping; use of contact helmets to treat **plagiocephaly,** but not craniosynostosis, is contemporary application of skull molding
6. **Deforming forces** appear to have much greater impact on lower than upper extremity development
   a. Much greater prenatal uterine constraint experienced by the legs
   b. Lower extremities carry the body weight and maintain erect position during growth, placing much more stress on them and increasing tendency for malalignment over time
   c. Anatomy of hip joint with multiple axes of motion but little osseous stability is disadvantage for a weightbearing joint; ankle also has multiple joint axes, but good osseous stability compared to the hip
   d. Influence of malalignment forces on adjacent joints is greater in a closed kinetic chain

Examples of joint or bone malalignment (see Tables 1.6 to 1.8)

1. **Scoliosis and kyphoscoliosis** may develop prenatally due to wedge-shaped vertebral bodies or fused vertebrae
   a. More commonly related to asymmetrical muscle pull or lack of support of the trunk related to paralysis
   b. Contributing conditions are cerebral palsy, spina bifida, spinal muscle atrophy, poliomyelitis, osteogenesis imperfecta, and muscular dystrophies

Table 1.6. Typical Progression of Femoral Neck-Shaft Angle

Age	Mean	Range of Values
4 months' gestational age	140°	130–150
8 months' gestational age	128°	112–143
birth	135°	118–144
1–3 years	145°	131–148
4–5 years	135°	123–143
9–13 years	135°	121–148
15–17 years	130°	121–148
adult	125°	114–140

2. **Coxa valga:** increased angle of inclination of the femoral neck relative to the femoral shaft in the frontal plane
   a. Approximately 135° at birth
   b. Decreases with weightbearing and balanced muscle pull under normal circumstances to 125–130° by adulthood
   c. Abnormal stresses negatively influence acetabular development and contribute to increased incidence of hip dislocation
3. **Coxa vara:** decreased angle of inclination of the femoral neck relative to the femoral shaft in the frontal plane to < 125°; decreased pressure on acetabulum and increased bending stress on femoral neck leads to predisposition for femoral neck fractures and slipped capital femoral epiphysis
4. **Femoral anteversion:** anterior rotation (version or torsion), in the transverse plane, of the upper femur relative to the femoral condyles
   a. Normally exceeds 25° in the infant and young child
   b. Decreases to 15° in the adult with growth, balanced muscle pull, and weightbearing
   c. Infantile anteversion frequently maintained in the growing child with spastic cerebral palsy, contributing to in-toeing gait pattern

Table 1.7. Typical Progression of Femoral Version

Age	Mean	Range
4 months' gestational age	12° degrees anteversion	15 retro–30° anteversion
8 months' gestational age	28°	10–55° anteversion
birth	30°	15–55°
1–3 years	35°	20–50°
4–5 years	25°	19–38°
10–12 years	25°	10–35°
13–20 years	14°	5 retro–33° anteversion
adult	15°	25 retro–35° anteversion

Table 1.8. Typical Progression of Tibiofemoral Angle

Age	Mean	Range of Values
birth	16° varus	34 varus–0 valgus
6 months	12° varus	
1 year	10° varus	21 varus–13 valgus
20 months	0°	
2 years	2° valgus	20 varus–20 valgus
30 months	8° valgus	
3 years	10° valgus	13 varus–19 valgus
4 years	9° valgus	4 varus–17 valgus
5 years	7° valgus	0 varus–11 valgus
6 years	6° valgus	0 varus–11 valgus
7–13 years	5° valgus	0 varus–14 valgus

   d. In absence of spasticity, often associated with compensatory lateral tibial torsion
   e. In presence of spasticity, often associated with medial tibial torsion, ankle pronation, and difficulty achieving functional hip external rotation
5. **Femoral retroversion:** posterior rotation, in the transverse plane, of upper femur relative to femoral condyles to <15° anteversion
   a. Rarely a drawback for the average person, although occasionally accompanied by compensatory medial tibial torsion
   b. Advantage for ballet dancers desiring hip external rotation
6. **Genu valgus, varus:** increased lateral (valgus) or medial (varus) knee (tibiofemoral) angulation in the frontal plane
   a. May be due to hamstring, quadriceps, hip adductor, or hip abductor weakness or spasticity
   b. Frequent contributors are joint disease or loss of ligamentous integrity, rather than muscle imbalance
7. **Medial, lateral tibial rotation:** tibia rotates in relation to femur at the knee joint
   a. Very common in neonates
   b. Often due to ligamentous laxity, but can result from unbalanced muscle pull, especially medial rotation associated with medial hamstring spasticity and/or ankle pronation, hip anteversion
   c. Tibial rotation more common than tibial torsion in children with spina bifida
8. **Medial, lateral tibial torsion:** rotation within the tibial shaft leading to spiral development of the bone; medial torsion typically associated with muscle imbalance of knee-ankle and ankle-foot muscles, especially in children with spastic cerebral palsy
9. **Ankle and foot deformities** associated with muscle imbalance are extensive; see Table 3.1 on Joint Deformations

ORIGINS AND EMERGENCE OF MOTOR BEHAVIORS (SEE TABLES 1.9 TO 1.11)

Origins of motor behavior are embryonic.

1. Fetal movements clearly visible by 7–8 weeks' gestational age using high-resolution ultrasonography
   a. Movement patterns arise spontaneously and are not reflexive
   b. Anatomical maturation of the arms and legs proceeds cephalocaudally, but movements in the upper extremity do not predate those in the lower extremities
   c. No gender-related differences in fetal movements
   d. Myelination does not precede the emergence of prenatal movement and is not required for it to occur
2. **Premature** infants: born less than 36 weeks' gestational age
   a. Infants born < 36 weeks' gestational age and weighing about 2500 g represent 5% of all births; 1% of these infants weigh < 1500 g
   b. Postural and motor development of premature infants often different from full term infants during the first year
   c. **Factors impeding motor development** can include infant respiratory distress syndrome **(IRDS),** bronchopulmonary dysplasia **(BPD),** retinopathy of prematurity **(ROP),** intraventricular hemorrhage **(IVH),** periventricular leukomalacia **(PVL),** hyperbilirubinemia, and necrotizing enterocolitis **(NEC)**

Emergence of motor behaviors is characterized by structural and schedule variation.

1. **Cultural variations**
   a. Biological differences and caregiving practices contribute to differences in motor development that are particularly apparent during the first 2 years
   b. Infants of African heritage demonstrate gross motor acceleration
      - Motorically very responsive at birth; high muscle tone and unusually good head control during a pull-to-sit maneuver
      - Caregiving practices emphasize antigravity activities and stimulatory handling
   c. Infants of Asian heritage and some American Indian infants have relaxed developmental motor progression
      - Low emotional and muscle tone at birth, little frustration, and high tolerance for disquieting events
      - Caregiving practices encourage calmness in the infant
   d. Motor development of Caucasian and Hispanic infants generally between those of infants of African or Asian heritage
   e. Developmental differences attributed to cultural variation may be result of maternal or infant malnutrition
2. **Varied locomotor progressions** exist in infants and children in the same cultural group

Table 1.9. Comparison of Preterm and Full-term Postural and Motor Development

	Full-term	Preterm
4 weeks	Posture dominated by flexion Sitting: head in midline, arms by side	Posture dominated by extension Sitting: *very* rounded back and forward head position
8 weeks	Prone suspension: head in line with body	Prone suspension: complete flexion
4 months	Sitting with slight support: back straight, head erect	Needs more support in sitting, scapular retraction, forward head position, fisting
5 months	Prone on elbows: shoulder-scapula co-contraction, back extension with head upright	Difficulty pushing up and maintaining position; minimal back extension with head in line with trunk
6 months	Prone: weight on pelvis; lateral weight shifting during reaching in prone	Prone: weight taken on lower rib cage, minimal head righting
	Supine: sufficient abdominal and LE strength to lift pelvis, activate abdominals, reach for feet	Supine: no lifting of pelvis, reach for knees, abdominals do not stabilize pelvis
	Rolling with rotation supine to prone	Emergence of lateral righting, may roll with hyperextension of back
	Sitting: back straight, arms free, beginning to shift weight laterally in preparation for transitions	Prop sitting: back rounded, lack of lateral weight shift
	Bears weight in standing with wide base, grading of flexion and extension	Minimal weight bearing: often up on toes, stiffening of LE or extremely wide base

Table 1.9. continued

	Full-term	Preterm
9 months	Standing: base of support narrows, rotates trunk, arms by side	Standing: lordosis, wide base of support, shoulder retraction
	Crawls on all fours, trunk even	If crawling, wide base between knees, lordosis, shoulder elevation
12 months	Stands alone, walks (at least with help); base of support narrow	Stands with support, base of support narrow, arms out to side, stiffening of LE, lordosis
	Transitions in and out of sitting using lateral weight shifting	Difficulty with transitions due to poor lateral weight shifting

a. About 12% of children do not crawl or creep before attaining typical ambulation
b. Bottom scooting and commando crawling are strategies utilized by children having no evidence of motor impairment

PSYCHOSOCIAL AND EMOTIONAL DEVELOPMENT

Infants and children are **more than kinetic performers.**

1. Movement capability may be a therapeutic priority, but other interdependent attributes also influence child's performance
   a. **Temperament**
      - Biologically based, consistent over time
      - Includes child's motor activity level, daily rhythm, moods, adaptability, social interaction, and environmental responsivity
      - May be a critical influence on child's overt behaviors and responses to intervention strategies

   b. **Attachment**
      - Parent-child attachment basis for overall societal cohesion
      - Child's attachment status influences how child deals with his or her environment
      - Most information available on **maternal**-infant attachment
        - **Securely attached** infants use the mother's position as a home base from which to explore enthusiastically and learn
        - **Anxious-avoidant** infants explore the environment with minimal or no contact with the mother

Table 1.10. Emergence of Motor Behaviors to One Year of Age

Age	Prone	Supine	Sitting	Hand and Arm	Locomotion	Atypical Behaviors
10-15 weeks' gestational age fetus				Isolated extremity movements by 11–13 weeks; hands to face, thumb in mouth, sucking by 15 weeks	Fetal displacement via full–body rotation around the umbilicus; climbing activities relative to uterine wall	Fetal akinesia sequence due to external factors such as crowding, insufficient amniotic fluid, or intrinsic neuromuscular disease
17-18 weeks' gestational age fetus				Lower and upper extremity motor development concurrent	Vigorous extensor thrusts against uterine wall reposition fetus and encourage maternal incontinence	Highly symmetrical, stereotypical movements lacking extremity dissociation from each other and from the trunk
20 weeks' gestational age fetus				Wide arcs of arm movement; creeping/crawling apparent	Period of greatest fetal motility, then decreases due to growth, increased sleep cycles	Absent or limited fetal propulsive movements associated with breech position, joint contractures

Table 1.10. continued

Age	Prone	Supine	Sitting	Hand and Arm	Locomotion	Atypical Behaviors
24-week premature infant	Sleeping most of time, froglike position and very low muscle tone	Extensor bias, low tone, froglike position, stays where positioned	Unstable physiologic responses, especially cardiorespiratory, discourage handling	Jittery movements, especially distal; elicited responses are primarily avoidant or disorganized	No evidence of locomotion; occasional, isolated extremity movement	Viability and cardiorespiratory capability primary concerns, rather than motor performance
30-week premature infant	Longer periods of alertness; minimal quadrupedal effort	Extensor bias; disorganized kicking	No ability to right in sitting; still some physiological instability	Hand swiping, hand-to-mouth self-comforting movements	Quadrupedal efforts in prone may result in scooting to corner of isolette	Very low muscle tone, little or no spontaneous movement; cardiorespiratory instability
35-week premature infant	Head elevates to bob and clear face; quadrupedal movements	Temporal linkage emerging among hip, knee, ankle during kicking	No evidence of self-support or righting in supported sitting	Hand-to-face and to-mouth movements better controlled	Prone infant may move from center toward corner or side of isolette	Poor or absent sucking, little spontaneous movement; inability to interact with caregivers

Table 1.10. continued

Age	Prone	Supine	Sitting	Hand and Arm	Locomotion	Atypical Behaviors
Neonatal period (full-term infant)	Head elevates to clear face and reposition it facing opposite direction; clear flexion bias in trunk and extremities	Head rotates fully in either direction, often while tracking object; head statically faces one side, usually right, but comes to midline with arousal	Head may bob while in kyphotic, supported sitting position; head position typically forward flexion; rapidly finds nipple and flexes toward it	Hands fisted much of time, arms often held snug to body; very strong elicited grasp, but hands open fully; isolated digital motions	Prone infant may achieve snug body placement against side of isolette after being placed in center; supine to sidelying roll in some infants; neonatal stepping	Hands fisted, absence of isolated digital movement; head always positioned to the side; inability to clear face in prone or exaggerated head elevation; head thrusting may impede finding nipple, sucking
1 month	Quadrupedal movements; head elevation linked with minimal forearm support	Reciprocal kicking alternates with symmetrical kicking	Shoulders and head remain quite forward but lower back more extended; head in line with trunk for short intervals	Pre-reaching efforts depend on body position and are linked with visual gaze on an object; spontaneous grasp and release	Rolls from side to back; may be able to relocate in prone when in crib	Difficulty flexing legs under body, limited arcs of extremity movement; absence of reciprocal leg movements, no evidence of grasp and release

Table 1.10. continued

Age	Prone	Supine	Sitting	Hand and Arm	Locomotion	Atypical Behaviors
2–3 months	Elbows in line with shoulders for forearm support; lateral weightshifting culminates in roll to supine (3 mo.)	Hand-foot play contributes to pelvic elevation off support surface	Midline head alignment in most all positions, minimal head lag during pull-to-sit; propped sitting may be emerging	Sufficient eye-hand coordination for reach, grasp and sustained shaking of a rattle; finger play in mouth	Pivot-prone rotation beginning, may achieve a 25–30° arc	Inability to right head during pull-to-sit maneuver or elevate pelvis to bring feet to hands; head elevation in prone to 90° is suspect
4–5 months	Weightshifting to free and reach with one hand; trunk elevation with elbow extension may be complete, followed by release to rock pelvis	Alternates feet to mouth and bridging; attempts roll from supine to side with leg or arm leading	Static ring sitting emerging, up to complete independence; attempts lateral weightshift to load one arm and grasp toy with other	Arms extend fully up in supine to reach to midline for bimanual toy play; palmar grasp of cube if seated securely; bimanual toy play all positions	Pivot-prone rotation well established; alternates between pivot-prone and quadruped; may attempt rocking in quadruped and pushing backwards	Lateral weightshifting difficult to free hand for reaching in prone; unable to extend arms fully and toward midline in supine; kyphotic sitting position, unable to sit erect

Table 1.10. continued

Age	Prone	Supine	Sitting	Hand and Arm	Locomotion	Atypical Behaviors
6–7 months	Rocks on hands and knees; transitions to sitting, kneeling emerging; pushes backward in prone	Feet to chin or mouth easily, rapid roll to prone, vigorous sit-up with external support	Static sitting with toy manipulation; weightshifting, lateral and anterior arm support	Grips cup or bottle with two hands; rakes for raisin; ulnar-palmar and radial-palmar grasp emerging	Forward propulsion, mainly with arms if abdomen on ground, or crawling with abdomen elevated (12% of AVERAGE children don't crawl)	Inability to sit erect without support; inability to achieve midline hand position in supine or sitting; no evidence of lateral or forward propulsion
8–9 months	Fluid transitions in/out of sitting to quadruped; may begin to pull to stand with external support	Resistant to remaining in supine; diaper change often a battle; easily lifts head	Rests on one arm out of midline while manipulating toy with other; anterior, lateral protective reactions present; posterior emerging	Controlled release; cube passed hand to hand, removed from cup; radial digital grasp with thumb, 2 fingers; scoots on bottom with toy in hand	Crawling/creeping well established if present; may pull to stand with external support, but needs rescue to get down or abruptly drops	No transition from commando crawl or bunny-hop to reciprocal locomotion; W-sit only or preferred sitting position

Table 1.10. continued

Age	Prone	Supine	Sitting	Hand and Arm	Locomotion	Atypical Behaviors
10–11 months	Pulls to standing by rolling up over feet; may begin to achieve stand by ½ kneeling; bounces in standing		Rotates or pivots while sitting to reach a toy; fast, smooth transitions to prone or supine	Thumb-finger inferior pincer grasp to pick up a raisin emerging	Sidesteps or cruises with external support; may start walking independently if poor crawler	Inability to transition among sitting positions or to achieve long-sitting due to insufficient hamstring length; mass grasp pattern
1 year	Transitions from prone to standing through ½ kneel; knee release to support smooth descent from standing		Wide variety of sitting positions includes side-sitting and choices to support manipulative activities	Bangs 2 cubes; ability to give and take a toy well established; rolls a ball away	Transitions among support surfaces; independent walking with high guard arms and wide support base unless very capable crawler/creeper	Inappropriate trunk and extremity stiffness, or laxity; instability; poor coordination may prevent hands-knees locomotion and emergence of standing

Table 1.11. Emergence of Motor and Adaptive Behaviors 1–5 Years of Age

Age	Gross Motor	Fine Motor	Self-Help or Communication	Sphincter	Locomotion	Atypical Behaviors
13–14 months	Sustained standing without external support; stoops to pick up object and regains standing	Holds two cubes in same hand, builds 2 cube tower, grasps with thumb opposing first 2 fingers	Points at desired objects or people; may kiss own face in mirror; says 2–3 words, plays pat-a-cake		Most children prefer walking; 12 months average age for independent walking; climbs into adult chairs	Absence of transition from bottom scooting, bunny hopping, or sequential rolling to more mature forms of locomotion
15–16 months	Arm position while walking is mid- or low-guard; creeps up steps or walks up with external support	Builds tower with 3 cubes; hurls objects to floor from table or high chair; flings ball with extensor thrust	Takes off shoes, pulls at socks; holds arm for sleeve, foot for sock; self-feeding with fingers, drinks from cup	May tell mother or father if pants are wet or soiled	Walks backward few steps, stoops & recovers easily; carries object while walking; starting to stand from floor	If onset of walking has not occurred, screen for delays in other areas to determine if need exists for in-depth assessment

Table 1.11. continued

Age	Gross Motor	Fine Motor	Self-Help or Communication	Sphincter	Locomotion	Atypical Behaviors
17–18 months	Carries or pulls an object while walking; creeps down steps; steps on ball positioned for kicking; tries steps using rail	Turns book pages several at a time; scribbles; builds tower with 3–4 cubes; takes pegs from board and attempts to replace	Takes off socks, anticipates shirt removal with arm placement, tugs at shirt, pants; 20-word vocabulary	May be dry for several hours during the day	Base of support almost equivalent to width of pelvis; running not well coordinated or with arm reciprocation	18 months ceiling age for onset of independent ambulation; if not present, refer for comprehensive evaluation for developmental delay
20–22 months	Walks up steps with step-to pattern and external one-hand support; easily stoops and recovers	Builds 5–6 cube tower; places pellet in bottle inconsistently; separates pop beads	Identifies some body parts; pulls adults to point out objects; uses fork	May consent to sit on potty with book and acknowledge presence of outcome in potty seat	Running speed and fluidity increasing; tries to jump off bottom step; descends steps with step-to pattern inconsistently with external support	Base of support much wider than pelvis often associated with low muscle tone, poor balance, and coordination; base of support too narrow associated with high tone, poor balance

Table 1.11. continued

Age	Gross Motor	Fine Motor	Self-Help or Communication	Sphincter	Locomotion	Atypical Behaviors
2 years	Kicks small ball forward; throws ball overhand for 5 feet; jumps off low step; 2-foot jump from floor emerging	Builds 6–7 cube tower; turns book pages singly; turns doorknobs, puts on shoes, socks, pulls pants up and down	Uses spoon or fork with little spillage; combines words to phrases; washes and dries hands; identifies 6 body parts	Wakes from naps dry; may be dry during the day, dry at night if awakened to urinate before parents go to bed	Ascends stairs alone, step-to pattern; attempts foot-over-foot with adult support; descends steps with step-to pattern	Walking pattern unresponsive to level changes; poor leg and trunk alignment, insecure balance leading to many falls
30 months	Jumps off step with 1 foot leading, 2 feet emerging; jumps off floor with 2 feet; can imitate walking on tiptoes; mounts tricycle	8 cube tower; pours well one glass to another; imitates straight, horizontal, and circular strokes with marker; tripod grip starts	Identifies all major body parts; finds armholes in coat consistently; may help to put things away; identifies objects from pictures	Climbs onto toilet; may be relatively independent with removal, replacing of clothing; help needed for wiping	Often ascends steps reciprocally; reciprocal step descent emerging with help; jumps off surfaces achieved by climbing (scares parent!)	Tentative in most/all gross motor activities; difficulty determining body placement for mounting ride-on toys; lack of emergence of accommodating grasp for smaller objects

Table 1.11. continued

Age	Gross Motor	Fine Motor	Self-Help or Communication	Sphincter	Locomotion	Atypical Behaviors
3 years	Jumps off step to land with 2 feet; easily propels riding vehicle with feet on floor, may be pedaling; stands on 1 foot briefly	9 cube tower; unbuttons buttons; imitates cross-stroke with marker; attempts scissor cut; imitates block bridge building; hand preference emerging	Understands turn-taking; practices counting; may be independent in dressing except for tying shoes and buttoning; uses rotary motions for washing and drying hands	May be independent for toileting during day, dry during the night; may need assistance with clothing or wiping; may not yet be dry through the night	Early reciprocal arm motion during running; jumps over 1–2 inch objects on floor; descends steps with no external support, step-to; kicks ball inconsistently; arms anticipate arrival of ball	Reluctance to help with or complete dressing; unable to mount, dismount or sustain any rotary motion on the pedals of a riding toy; base of support may remain abnormally wide or narrow, indicative of ongoing balance or tonal responsivity problems
42 months	Mounts, pedals and dismounts several types	10 cube tower; strings & unstrings	Attempts and sometimes succeeds with button-		Kicks various balls inconsistently; runs to ball, then	Response times insufficient to succeed at catching a ball

Table 1.11. continued

Age	Gross Motor	Fine Motor	Self-Help or Communication	Sphincter	Locomotion	Atypical Behaviors
	of three-wheel riding vehicles; stands on 1 foot for > 3 seconds, begins hopping on 1 foot	beads based on size; builds bridges using blocks; removes bottle cap to check contents	ing; may help set and clear the table; asks many questions		kicks emerging; may jump with 2 feet several times in succession	or soft object; skills requiring static and dynamic single leg stability, such as kicking, hopping, standing on one leg not emerging
4 years	Rotation of body follows forward projection of ball; several hops in succession on 1 foot; stands and walks on tiptoes if so inclined	Dynamic tripod pencil grip in some children; cross-strokes with marker; attempts to trace line; clear hand preference	Understands notion of responsibility; negotiates with adults roles and responsibilities; may be independent in bathing	Toilet independence in majority; small percentage of children with no motor or cognitive delay still not dry during night	Few children ride two-wheel bike, many use training wheels; running fluid with strong emergence of upper arm reciprocation	Skills requiring moderate to maximal balance challenges such as climbing and jumping off heights not attempted; catching, kicking balls difficult; hand preference ambiguous

Table 1.11. continued

Age	Gross Motor	Fine Motor	Self-Help or Communication	Sphincter	Locomotion	Atypical Behaviors
54 months	Catches ball by fluid accommodation of arm as ball approaches, elbows may be at sides; throws ball to another person 8–10 feet away; jumps 2–3″ off floor	Folds sheet of paper in half; cuts large square from paper sheet; drops raisins or pellets into small bottle moderately quickly	Unlaces shoes, laces 2–3 holes, imitates looping lace; buttons and unbuttons; acts out fantasies with imaginary characters		Several steps on curb, wall or beam without falling; runs to scoop up ball and throw it; reaches for overhead trapeze to lift body weight off support surface	Difficulty with skills requiring asymmetrical body positioning or dissociated extremity movements, i.e. rotatory arm or leg movements, throwing with one arm, jumping from one leg

Table 1.11. continued

Age	Gross Motor	Fine Motor	Self-Help or Communication	Sphincter	Locomotion	Atypical Behaviors
5 years	Jumps forward and sideways with two-foot takeoff, two-foot landing emerging; jumps over object 6–8″ from floor; throws ball to hit target at 10 ft	Dynamic tripod grip; drawing of simple shapes, letters, or numbers may be attempted; places small pegs in pegboard and removes them easily; winds string on spool	Ample vocabulary to communicate with adults and children in familiar situations; negotiates with playmates in complex play situations		Many children solo on a two-wheel bike, roller skates, based on opportunities for practice; fluid running, arm reciprocation well established; broad jump emerging	Difficulty mounting or pedaling any ride-on toy; often cannot imitate a motor act after seeing another child complete it; base of support wider than pelvis; cannot catch ball; fist grip rather than tripod grip of marker or pencil

- ◦ **Anxious-resistant** infants are passive and show great reluctance to separate from the mother; high correlation with low birth weight, low Apgar scores, motor immaturity, and self-regulatory problems

c. **Motivation**
- Contemporary view: child is an active seeker of stimulation, motivated to explore and gain environmental mastery, not just passively respond to physiological needs
- Basis for goal-oriented behavior
- Nurtured by responses to infant's earliest attempts to interact with the environment; child learns that outcomes are contingent upon his or her initiation
- Child's self-perception of limited influence on environmental outcomes may be basis for lack of motivation

d. **Cognition**
- Not equivalent to performance on an intelligence test; basis for child's problem-solving abilities in multiple domains; infant intelligence tests unreliable predictors
- Highly dependent on other aspects of development such as temperament and motivation
- "Looking smart:" assessment of cognitive ability may be inaccurately based on appearance
- Catch-up potential available up to 6 years of age following remediation of early, adverse, environmental circumstances

Developmental Perspectives (see Tables 1.12 and 1.13)

1. **Affective development: T. Berry Brazelton**
   a. Boston pediatrician who transformed infant assessment from stimulus-response maneuvers to a consideration of infant abilities
   b. Documented that neonates are socially interactive individuals who demonstrate their competencies when state is considered
2. **Cognitive development: Jean Piaget**
   a. Systematically recorded observations of children's (his, mostly) cognitive behavior; his findings are now confirmed in societies all over the world
   b. Organized cognitive development into a sequence of ordinal stages from the infant's need to directly interact with the environment **(sensorimotor stage)** to individual's ability to manipulate abstract concepts in the absence of direct experience **(formal operational stage)**
   c. Viewed child as acting on the environment and inferred cognition from motor behaviors observed in younger nonverbal children
   d. Basic premise is that children's mental representations of the world become more sophisticated in proportion to their widening radius of experience

3. **Child development in the context of family: Anna Freud**
   a. Influenced by father, Sigmund, who explored relationship of early childhood to subsequent development of psychopathology
   b. Main contribution is influence of family dynamics on child development and critical need to view child in the context of family
4. **Child development in the context of society: Erik Erikson**
   a. Expanded Anna Freud's emphasis on family interaction to human development in the context of cultural influences on the individual
   b. Developed an ordinal sequence for psychosocial growth based on progression through specific critical junctions, outcomes of which influenced subsequent behavioral responses
   c. Applied concept of **epigenetic** development: individual's personality forms as ego progresses through developmental stages

Table 1.12. Piagetian Stages of Cognitive Development

Stage	Sub-stages	Description
I. Sensorimotor Stage (approximately birth–2 years)	A. Reflex stage	Primitive life-sustaining behaviors present at birth quickly adapt to experience; tracking, thumb-sucking, orienting to sound
	B. Organization of percepts and habits	Infant learning contingency awareness: effect of actions on the environment
	1. Primary circular reactions (birth–8 months)	Influence of one action on another action confined to the infant's body
	2. Secondary circular reactions (8–10 months)	Infant's action on the environment generates a repetitive circuit; begins to modify behavior to test and change environmental responses
	3. Tertiary circular reactions (11 months or more)	Infant links together isolated behaviors that were secondary circular reactions into a chain; continually varies behaviors to test environment
	C. Sensorimotor or practical intelligence	Infant uses direct experience, principally manipulatory, to gain knowledge of the world; incorporates objects in the environment into action schemes
II. Preparation for and Organization of Concrete Operations	A. Pre-operational Stage (approximately 2–7 years of age)	Mental representation linked with language Child is focused on perceptual and spatial properties of objects Egocentricity Inability to understand conservation of number, mass, or volume

Table 1.12. continued

Stage	Sub-stages	Description
	B. Concrete Operational Stage (7–11 years of age)	Child now understands permanence of matter through transformations: Conservation of volume: 2 shapes of modeling clay same volume Conservation of number: 2 rows of coins different distance apart same # Conservation of weight: 2 shapes of modeling clay same weight Conservation of continuous quantity: same volume of water in 2 containers Child can order objects, put them into a 1:1 correspondence, and conserve equivalence with changes in physical arrangement
III. Formal Operations (approximately age 12 years–adulthood)		Can generalize to novel situations without direct experience Trial-and-error behavior utilized for generating and testing hypotheses Flexible, abstract thinking unrelated to direct experience Ability to imagine many possibilities inherent in one situation

Table 1.13. Erikson's Epigenetic Stages of Human Development

Age	Stage	Critical Issue	Related Factors
Birth–2 years	Infancy	Trust versus Mistrust	Consistent care Inadequate or inconsistent care
2–3 years	Early childhood	Autonomy versus Doubt or Shame	Freedom to explore, try skills Overprotection or lack of support leads to self-doubt
4–5 years	Preschool	Initiative versus Guilt	Freedom, direction Restriction
6–12 years	School Age	Industry versus Inferiority	Freedom Limitation and criticism
13–18 years	Adolescence	Identity versus Role confusion	Integration of sense of self Inability to establish stability in gender role or occupation
18–25 years	Young adulthood	Intimacy versus Isolation	Devotion to another Combative or competitive personal relations
25–50 years	Middle adulthood	Generativity versus Self-absorption	Guidance for next generation Isolation, possibly due to illness
>50 years	Mature adulthood	Integrity versus Despair, Disgust	Acceptance of one's life Cannot recover lost opportunities

2 / Measurement

Toby M. Long

Therapists have long recognized the importance of accurate measurement in determining the needs of children with developmental disabilities, musculoskeletal dysfunction, and other conditions. As with other areas of pediatric physical therapy, there has been an evolution in the types of measurements taken on children throughout the years. Whereas therapists used to rely on clinical observations to make intervention decisions, they now use standardized tests and developmental checklists to determine deviation from age-expected norms. Presently physical therapists are moving toward a functional outcome approach to assess children in determining intervention needs.

Contributing to these shifts in focus has been an appreciation of the advantages and disadvantages of measurement and the information which can be obtained from the measurement process. The purpose of this chapter is to provide a basic understanding of the measurement process, to introduce the reader to a variety of measurement tools, and to outline clinical measurement strategies commonly used in pediatric physical therapy. In relation to the standardized measures discussed, readers are advised to refer to the test manuals and to experienced test administrators prior to administering and interpreting a standardized measure.

MEASUREMENT

Measurement, the process of quantifying characteristics of an individual, involves three components: characteristics of the individual that the examiner wants to measure must be clearly defined, a system of observations must be developed, and a set of rules turning observations into quantifiable units must be devised.

Measurement should follow the need for information to determine developmental status, musculoskeletal status, cardiopulmonary status, etc., of a child in order to: (1) diagnose, (2) determine placement, (3) plan intervention, (4) determine progress, (5) determine efficacy of programming, and (6) do research.

Standardized tests are specific measuring instruments that (1) adhere to specific instructions that guide the administration of each item and (2) possess sound psychometric characteristics.

Psychometric characteristics

1. Norm-referenced vs. criterion-referenced (Table 2.1)
2. Validity—degree to which a meaningful interpretation can be inferred from a measurement

Table 2.1. Standardized Measurement

Norm-Referenced	Criterion-Referenced
Standard point scores	Cut-off scores
Compares individual performance against group performance	Compares performance against a described standard
May or may not be related to therapeutic/instructional content	Content specific
Normal distribution of scores desired	Variability of scores not obtained, mastery of skills desired
Maximizes differences among individuals	Discriminates between successive performances of one individual
Requires diagnostic skills of examiner	Provides information to plan therapy/instruction
Not sensitive to effects of therapy or instruction	Sensitive to effects of instruction
Not concerned with task analysis	Depends on task analysis
Summative	Formative

a. Content: how well items of measurement instrument represent theoretical basis of trait to be studied
b. Construct: how well instrument accurately represents theoretical basis of trait to be studied
c. Criterion-related: how well instrument correlates with another instrument purporting to measure same construct or trait
   - Concurrent: two instruments purporting to measure a specific trait administered simultaneously correlate with one another
   - Predictive: one instrument given at a specific time correlates with another instrument purporting to measure same trait at a later time.

3. Reliability—degree to which instrument produces consistent/repeatable results
   a. Internal consistency: the degree to which all items of test are measuring the same concept
   b. Inter-rater: degree of agreement among two or more testers of the same test given to the same individual (percent agreement, ICC)
   c. Standard error of measurement: used to develop a range of probable scores around the obtained score that is likely to indicate the child's "true" ability level on that test
   d. Test-retest: correlation between two administrations of the same test to the same individual on two separate occasions
4. Sensitivity: ability of the instrument to detect dysfunction/abnormality (positive finding)

5. Specificity: ability of the instrument to detect normality (negative finding)
6. Scores: meaningful only in relation to stated referent (Fig. 2.1); provide information on how well a child performs compared to a population; norms: based on normal distribution of scores on a large sample of the population (normative sample)
   - Percentiles: ranking based on the percentage of individuals in the normative sample who received a score above or below the score received
   - Stanine (standard nine): single digit score (1–9) based on mean and standard deviation of the group
   - Age/grade equivalent: represents how well the average child at a particular age or grade performed on the particular test given; can be misleading, especially grade equivalents

CATEGORIES OF MEASUREMENT INSTRUMENTS

Screening

1. To identify the risk for dysfunction in specific categories of children
2. To detect the risk for dysfunction in an individual child
3. To formulate a register or monitoring system for children identified at risk
4. Usually done at regular intervals (i.e., yearly)

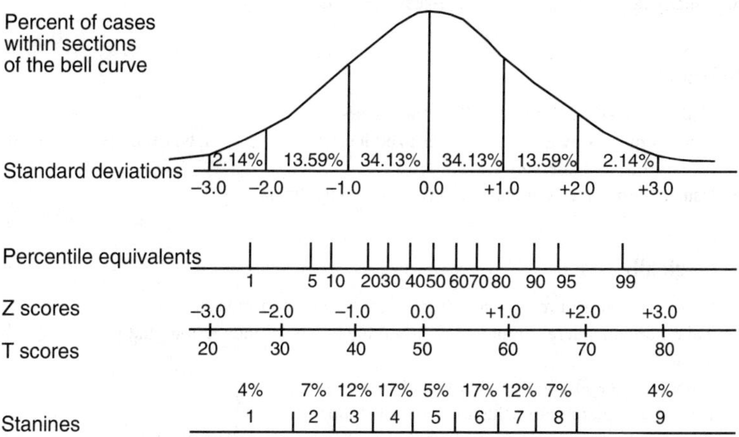

Figure 2.1. Relationship of frequently used standard scores to the bell curve.

Evaluation

1. To diagnose
2. To identify atypical development
3. To obtain baseline information on child's performance or status
4. To determine eligibility for service
5. Usually norm-referenced and/or formal
6. Usually done once or infrequently (i.e., triannually)

Assessment

1. To program plan
2. To delineate strengths, weaknesses, and needs across domains and environments
3. Often are criterion-referenced and/or informal
4. Done on an ongoing basis (i.e., within treatment)

CLASSES OF MEASUREMENT INSTRUMENTS (TABLE 2.1)

Formal

1. Child-centered (individual skill performance)
2. Sources of information: standardized; criterion- or norm-referenced instruments
3. Usually done at regular intervals (weekly, monthly, yearly, etc.)

Informal

1. Child-centered (individual skill performance)
2. Sources of information: nonstandardized instruments, checklists, developmental skill level forms, and interviews
3. Usually done on an ongoing basis (i.e., within treatment)

Ecologically Based

1. Child-environment relationship (functional activity performance)
2. Take into consideration physical environment, social interaction, and psychological status
3. Emphasis: adaptivity of the individual
4. Describes repertoire of behavior across domains
5. Sources of information: clinical ratings, anecdotal records, and inventories
6. Usually done on an ongoing basis and across environments

MEASUREMENT INSTRUMENTS FREQUENTLY USED BY PEDIATRIC PHYSICAL THERAPISTS (TABLE 2.3)

Developmental

These instruments are commonly used for diagnosis and are based on a maturational perspective. They attempt to assess an individual's skill development based on normative samples or accepted skill sequences. They represent the perspective that maturation is determined by genetic and biological factors and that these inherent factors are the central motivators for developmental change.

Table 2.2. Comparison of Classes

	Formal	Informal	Ecologically Based
Advantages	• Standardized • Established • Valid • Reliable	• Ease of administration • Obtain information on typical performance • Flexible to meet family needs	• Functional • Actual behaviors determine levels of development • Considers environment • Family can contribute control to the situation • Integration of domains • Can be linked to program planning • Child-directed
Disadvantages	• Lack of familiarity between tester and child • Restricted sample of behavior • Lacks family involvement	• Examiner bias • Lack of reliability • Lack of validity	• Restricted sample of behaviors • Prompting by partner can limit spontaneity of behavior • Environment may be detrimental

Table 2.3. Selected Measurement Instruments

Name	1. Perspective 2. Purpose 3. Class 4. Category	Areas Assessed	Population
Alberta Infant Motor Scale (AIMS), Piper, M, Darrah, J, Pinnell, L, Maguire, T, Byrne, P (1993)	1. Motor Performance 2. To assess postural control 3. Formal 4. Assessment, Screening	Postural control in supine, prone, sitting, standing	0–18 months
Amiel-Tison (Assessment for Gestational Age), Amiel-Tison, C, Grenier, A (1968)	1. Neurological 2. To determine gestational age 3. Formal 4. Evaluation	Passive tone Active tone Reflexes	Neonates
Assessment, Evaluation and Programming System for Infants and Children, Bricker, D (1993)	1. Behavioral 2. To determine skills and information child has and under what conditions they are used 3. Formal 4. Assessment	Fine motor, gross motor, adaptive, cognitive, social-communication, social	1 month–3 years
Assessment of Movement Activity in Infants, Haley, SM, Baryza, MJ, Coryell, J, Zilhenski, C (1989)	1. Motor performance 2. To measure change in children not walking 3. Formal 4. Assessment	Antigravity movement and posture	Infants

Psychometric Qualities	Clinical Implications	Source
Interrater reliability: very strong: .85–.99 concurrent validity: PDMS .85–.99, with BSID .84–.97	Minimal handling done by parent Quick Emphasis on components of motor milestones	Piper MC, Darrah J. *Motor assessment of the developing infant.* Philadelphia, PA: WB Saunders, 1993
No reliability provided	French angles commonly used in other tests	*Neurological evaluation of the newborn and the Infant.* New York: Masson
Interrater agreement: .70–.95 for domain, total test: .87 Test-retest reliability: .77–.95 for domain, total test: .88 Concurrent validity: Bayley Mental Scale .93, Motor Scale .88	Links measurement to specific curriculum Items on AEP's related to program goals	Paul H. Brookes Publishing Co, PO Box 10624, Baltimore, MD 21285-0624
Interrater reliability >.90 Summary scores discriminate between infants with and without disabilities	Videotape procedure limits handling of infant Attempts to quantify spontaneous movement	Research Training Center in Childhood Trauma and Rehabilitation, 750 Washington St, 75K-R2, Boston, MA 02111

Table 2.3. continued

Name	1. Perspective 2. Purpose 3. Class 4. Category	Areas Assessed	Population
Assessment of Preterm Infant Behavior (ABIP), Als H, Lester BM, Tronick EZ, Brazelton TB (1982)	1. Neurological/ Adaptive-transactive 2. To assess the individual behavioral organization of the preterm infant 3. Formal 4. Assessment	Physiologic, state, motor, attentional/interactive, regulatory	Preterm infants
Battelle Developmental Inventory (BDI), Newborg J, Stock JR, Wnek L (1984)	1. Behavioral 2. To determine level of development; to determine eligibility for educational intervention 3. Formal 4. Assessment	Personal-social, adaptive, motor, communication, cognition	1 month–9 years
Bayley Scales of Infant Development II; Bayley N (1993)	1. Developmental 2. To determine developmental status of infants 3. Formal 4. Evaluation	Cognitive, motor, behavior	0–42 months

Psychometric Qualities	Clinical Implications	Source
Interrater reliability: .90	Provides information on the infant's reaction to environmental changes Requires extensive training Primarily used as a research instrument Lengthy to administer	Fitzgerald H, Joyner MW, ed. *Theory & Research in Behavioral Pediatrics Vol I,* New York, NY: Plenum
Interrater, intrarater reliability range from .71–1.0; concurrent validity with PEDI .73 Small normative sample	Includes adaptations for children with disabilities Has screening tool Limited number of items in each domain	DLM Teaching Resources, One DLM Park, Allen, TX 75002
Test-retest reliability (all ages): mental .87, motor .78 (lower for younger ages and for behavioral record) Interrater reliability: mental .96, motor .75 Validity of mental scale with McCarthy Scales .79 for General Cognitive Index, with WPPSI .73 motor scale to GCI .45, to WPPSI .41	Predictive value is moderate in cognitive area, lower scores are more predictive Most widely used assessment in infant research	The Psychological Corporation, 555 Academic Ct., San Antonio, TX 78204-2498

Table 2.3. continued

Name	1. Perspective 2. Purpose 3. Class 4. Category	Areas Assessed	Population
Brigance Inventory of Early Development, Brigance AH (1978)	1. Developmental 2. To develop a comprehensive profile of developmental status 3. Formal 4. Assessment	Gross motor, fine motor, self-help, pre-speech, speech & language, general knowledge and comprehension, early academic	Birth–7 years
Bruininks-Oseretsky Test of Motor Proficiency, Bruininks R (1978)	1. Developmental 2. To assess motor performance 3. Formal 4. Evaluation	Gross motor, fine motor, upper limb coordination	41/2–141/2 years
The Carolina Curriculum for Infants and Toddlers with Special Needs (2nd ed.) Johnson-Martin NM, Jens KA, Attermeier SN & Hacker BJ (1991)	1. Behavioral 2. To determine level of performance across dimensions 3. Formal 4. Assessment	Cognition, communication, gross motor, fine motor, self-help	0–36 months
Chandler Movement Assessment of Infants: Screening Test (CMAI-ST), Chandler LS, Andrews M, Swanson M, Larson A	1. Neurological 2. To screen for movement disorders 3. Formal 4. Screening	Tone, primitive reflexes, automatic reactions, volitional movement	Infants below 12 months developmental level

Psychometric Qualities	Clinical Implications	Source
Criterion-referenced, no reliability data reported	Used in center-based programs to develop a comprehensive assessment of child across a wide variety of skills	Curriculum Associates, Inc., 5 Esquire 12d, North Billerica, MA 01862-2859
Test-retest reliability for battery composite .89, low for individual subtests	Short form available May be lengthy for younger children Item instructions may be too complex for younger children or individuals with language/cognitive disabilities	American Guidance Service, Publisher's Building, Circle Pines, MN 55014
Field-tested at 12 early intervention sites No psychometric data provided in manual	Criterion-referenced Gross motor section based on Rood Accompanied by a curriculum that is cross-referenced to measurement instrument	Paul H. Brookes Publishing Co, PO Box 10624, Baltimore, MD 21285-0624
Norms are being established for 2–12 month-olds	Scored from spontaneous movement	Infant Movement Research, PO Box 4631, Rolling Bay, WI 98061

Table 2.3. continued

Name	1. Perspective 2. Purpose 3. Class 4. Category	Areas Assessed	Population
DeGangi-Berk Test of Sensory Integration (TSI), DeGangi G, Berk R (1983)	1. Sensory 2. To assess underlying sensory motor mechanisms 3. Formal 4. Screening	Postural control, bilateral motor integration, reflex integration	3–5 years
Denver Developmental Screening Test II (DDST-II), Frankenburg WK, Dodds J, Archer P, et. al. (1990)	1. Developmental 2. To detect potential developmental problems 3. Formal 4. Screening	Gross motor, fine motor, language, personal-social	2 weeks–6 years
Developmental Test of Visual-Motor Integration (VMI), Beery KE, (1989)	1. Developmental 2. To determine skill level in the area of visual motor control 3. Formal 4. Screening	Visual-motor skills	2–15 years
Early Learning Accomplishment Profile (E-LAP), Glover ME, Preminger JL, Sanford AR (1978)	1. Developmental 2. To determine skill level through task analysis 3. Formal 4. Assessment	Gross motor, fine motor, cognitive, language, self-help, social-emotional	birth–36 months
Erhardt Developmental Prehension Assessment (EDPA), Erhardt RP (1982)	1. Developmental 2. To describe the components of comprehension 3. Formal 4. Assessment	Involuntary arm-hand patterns, primary voluntary movements, prewriting skills	birth–15 months

Psychometric Qualities	Clinical Implications	Source
Total test decision reliability: .93 Test-retest reliability: .85–.96 Interrater reliability: .80 Reflex subtest less reliable	Primarily used for screening of sensorimotor control	Western Psychological Services, 12031 Wilshire Blvd, Los Angeles, CA 90025
Interrater reliability: .99 Intrarater reliability: .90	Quick screening tool Prescreening developmental questionnaire (PDQ) completed by parents for DDST II is being developed	DDM, Inc., PO Box 6919, Denver, CO 80206-0914
Norm-referenced Interrater reliability: .93–.98 Test-retest: .63–.92 Validity with Bender-Gestalt: .41 to .82	Tends to underestimate skill level of children May be indicative of school readiness	Modern Curriculum Press, 13906 Prospect Road, Cleveland, OH 44136
Criterion-referenced No psychometric qualities provided	Tends to overestimate skill level Used often in early intervention programs	Kaplan School Supply Press, 1310 Lewisville Clemons Rd, Lewisville, NC 20023
Interrater reliability: 70.8–94.5% Lacks standardization	Administer to both hands Provides information linking assessment to treatment Based on a developmental sequence	*Developmental Hand Dysfunction: Theory, Assessment, Treatment.* RAMSCO Publishing Co, PO Box N, Laurel, MD 20707

Table 2.3. continued

Name	1. Perspective 2. Purpose 3. Class 4. Category	Areas Assessed	Population
Functional Independence Measure for Children (Wee-FIM), Granger C, Braun S, Griswood K, et al (1991)	1. Functional 2. Actual performance of child to indicate severity of disability 3. Formal 4. Evaluation	Self-care, sphincter control, mobility, locomotion, communication, social, cognition Gross motor, fine motor, language, personal-social, adaptive	6 months–7 years
Revised Gesell and Amatruda Developmental Neurological Exam, Knoblock H, Stevens F, Malone AF (1987)	1. Developmental 2. To determine developmental status 3. Formal 4. Evaluation	Gross motor, fine motor, language, personal-social, adaptive	4 weeks–5 years
Gross Motor Function Measure (GMFM), Russell D, Rosenbaum P, Garland C, et al (1990)	1. Behavioral 2. To evaluate change in function of children with cerebral palsy, to describe level of functioning, and to assist in treatment planning 3. Formal 4. Assessment	Lying and rolling, sitting, crawling and kneeling, standing, walking, and running and jumping	All ages; however, may be better suited for children 2–5 years

Psychometric Qualities	Clinical Implications	Source
Items selected and modified as needed from the FIM, content validity reported	Ease of administration Potential to provide continuity between pediatric and adult measures National database being established	Uniform Data System for Medical Rehabilitation, State University of New York, Research Foundation, 8Z Farber Hall, SUNY South Campus, Buffalo, NY 14214
Test-retest: .82 Predictive validity: .5–.85	Comprehensive, well respected measurement tool Some information gained from report	*Manual of Development: The Administration and Interpretation of Revised Gesell and Amatruda Developmental and Neurological Examination.* Gesell Developmental Materials, Inc., PO Box 272391, Houston, TX 77277-2391
Interrater and intrarater reliabilities of .87–above .92	Scoring based on how much of a task the child accomplishes Items more representative of skills developed below 3 years of age Excellent for treatment planning	Gross Motor Measures Group, Building 74, Room 29, Station 9, Hamilton, ON, Canada L8N 3Z5

Table 2.3. continued

Name	1. Perspective 2. Purpose 3. Class 4. Category	Areas Assessed	Population
Hawaii Early Learning Profile (HELP), Faruno S, O'Reilly K, Hosaka C, Inatsuka T, Allman T, Zeisloft-Falby B (1988)	1. Behavioral 2. To determine developmental level 3. Formal 4. Assessment	Cognition, language, gross motor, fine motor, social, self-help	0–36 months
Home Observation for Measurement of the Environment (HOME), Caldwell B (1984)	1. Adaptive-transactive 2. To determine how the home environment impacts the child 3. Informal 4. Assessment	Emotional and verbal responsiveness of parents, acceptance of child, organization of environment, provision of appropriate play materials, parental involvement, opportunities for stimulation	Birth–36 months
Infant Monitoring Questionnaires (IMQ), Squires J, Bricker D (1989)	1. Developmental 2. To determine developmental level through parent report 3. Formal 4. Screening	Communication, gross motor, fine motor, adaptive, personal-social	4–36 months
The Infant Motor Screen (IMS), Nickel R, Renken C, Gallenstein J (1989)	1. Neurological 2. To determine neurological status of preterm infants 3. Formal 4. Screening	Tone, primitive reflexes, automatic responses	Preterm infants at corrected ages 4–16 months

Psychometric Qualities	Clinical Implications	Source
Criterion-referenced	Administration and reference manual: *Inside HELP*, developed by Parks S (1992) *HELP at Home* is a book of home activity reproducible sheets consistent with the HELP	Vort Corp., PO Box 69880, Palo Alto, CA 94306
Interrater reliability: .90 Internal consistency .44–.89 Stability: .20–.60 Predictive validity: .38–.50	Effective for instructing families to develop a learning environment for child	Center for Child Development and Education, University of Arkansas at Little Rock, Little Rock, AR 72204
Test reliability high, interrater reliability high	Cost effective monitoring system for high-risk infants	Center on Human Development, University of Oregon, Eugene, OR 87043
Predictive validity for CP high Interrater agreement high	Easy-to-follow screening tool, takes into consideration degree of prematurity, quantitative scoring methods	Crippled Children's Division, The Oregon Health Sciences University, Clinical Services Bldg, Eugene, OR 87043

Table 2.3. continued

Name	1. Perspective 2. Purpose 3. Class 4. Category	Areas Assessed	Population
Infant Neurological International Battery (INFINIB), Ellison PH, Horn JL, Browning CA (1994)	1. Neurological 2. To determine neurological status of infant 3. Formal 4. Screening	Muscle tone, reflexes, automatic responses, head and trunk control	Neonates–9 months
Infant Toddler Scale for Every baby (ITSE), Miller, LJ (1992)	1. Developmental 2. To discriminate between normal and abnormal development 3. Informal 4. Screening	Cognitive, communication, physical, social-emotional, adaptive	3–42 months
Milani-Comparetti Motor Development Screening (M-C) Test, Stuberg W, et al (1987)	1. Developmental 2. To determine neuromotor maturation of infants 3. Formal 4. Screening	Reflexes, motor milestones	1–16 months
Miller Assessment of Preschoolers (MAP), Miller LJ (1982)	1. Developmental 2. To identify children with mild to moderate delays 3. Formal 4. Screening/assessment	Sensorimotor, cognitive, combined	2 years, 9 months–5 years, 8 months
Movement Assessment Battery for Children (Movement ABC), Henderson S, Sugden DA (1992)	1. Developmental 2. To identify and describe motor impairments 3. Formal 4. Assessment	Manual dexterity, balance, ball-handling, visual-motor	4–12 years

Psychometric Qualities	Clinical Implications	Source
Test-retest reliability of .95 Interrater: .97	May prove useful in infant follow-up programs	Therapy Skill Builders, PO Box 42050, Tucson, AZ 85733
No norms Test-retest reliability: .80–.91 Criterion-referenced	Administered by parent while therapist observes	Foundation for Knowledge in Development, 8101 E. Prentice Ave, Suite 518, Englewood, CO 80111
Intrarater reliability: .90–.93, Test-retest reliability high No cut-off scores	Quick, solid, reliable screening tools Interpretations of results must be made with caution	Meyer Children's Rehab. Institute, 444 South 44th St., Omaha, NE 68131-3795
Test-retest reliability: .81 Interrater reliability: .97 Correlation between MAP & WPPSI .27	Lengthy to administer Items very creative and maintain interest of child Does not provide age-equivalent scores Attempts to assess foundation skills such as postural control (basic sensorimotor tasks)	Psychological Corp, PO Box 839954, San Antonio, TX 78283-3954
Test-retest reliability: .75 Interrater reliability: .70	Quick Interesting, motivating items Picks up subtle problems	Psychological Corp, PO Box 839954, San Antonio, TX 78283-3954

Table 2.3. continued

Name	1. Perspective 2. Purpose 3. Class 4. Category	Areas Assessed	Population
Movement Assessment of Infants (MAI), Chandler LS, Swanson MW, Andrews MS (1980)	1. Neurological 2. To provide a uniform approach to the evaluation of high risk infants 3. Formal 4. Assessment	Muscle tone, reflexes, automatic reactions, volitional movement	0–12 months
Naturalistic Observation of Newborn Behavior (NONB), Als H (1981)	1. Behavioral 2. To develop a profile of infants' physiological and behavioral responses to environmental demands and caregiving 3. Formal 4. Assessment	State, autonomic responses, motor	Neonates–4 weeks post term
Neonatal Behavioral Assessment Scale (NBAS), Brazelton TB (1973)	1. Adaptive-transactive/Neurological 2. To determine interactive behavior and neuromotor status 3. Formal 4. Assessment	State, muscle tone, reflexes, interactive behavior	Birth–1 month
Neonatal Neurobehavioral Exam (NNE), Morgan A, Loch V, Lee V, Alday J (1988)	1. Neuromotor 2. To determine neurobehavioral status of infants 3. Formal 4. Evaluation	Tone, motor patterns, primitive reflexes, behavioral responses	Infants < 32 weeks' gestation–40 weeks' gestation

Psychometric Qualities	Clinical Implications	Source
Interrater reliability fair Test-retest reliability fair Poor predictive validity High rate of false positives	Lengthy, great deal of handling of the infant Risk profile for 4-month-old	Infant Movement Research, PO Box 4631, Rolling Bay, WI 18061
None available	Information gained through observation only	Neonatal Individualized Developmental Care and Assessment Program Training Materials, Neuro-behavioral Infant and Child Studies, Enders Ped Research Lab, Children's Hosp, Boston, MA
Interrater reliability: .90 Test-retest reliability: fair Predictive validity significant Percent agreement high Concurrent validity high	Provides a wealth of information on the individuality of infants Response to interaction Stresses state control	Clinics in Developmental Medicine No. 50, J.B. Lippincott Co., Philadelphia, PA 19105
Minimal amount of information Interrater reliability for full-term infants: .88 Predictive validity low for NNE & PDMS	Very quick to administer Lacks standardized testing procedures	Physical Therapy 68(9): 1352-1358

Table 2.3. continued

Name	1. Perspective 2. Purpose 3. Class 4. Category	Areas Assessed	Population
Neonatal Oral-Motor Assessment Scale (NOMAS), Braun MA, Palmer MM (1985)	1. Functional 2. To identify oral motor dysfunction in the neonate 3. Formal 4. Screening	Jaw and tongue patterns during nutritive and non-nutritive sucking	Neonate
Neurobehavioral Assessment of Preterm Infant (NAPI), Korner AF, Thom VA (1990)	1. Adaptive-transactive/Neurological 2. To determine neurobehavioral status of infants, determine effects of intervention, study infant development and individual differences 3. Formal 4. Assessment	State, behavior, reflexes, motor patterns, tone	32–42 weeks' gestation
The Neurologic Assessment of the Preterm and Full-term Newborn Infant, Dubowitz L, Dubowitz V (1981)	1. Neurological 2. To provide an evaluation of functional neurological status 3. Formal 4. Evaluation	Tone, posture, spontaneous movement, primitive reflexes, tendon reflexes	Infants 38–42 weeks' gestation
Neurological Exam of the Full Term Infant, Prechtl H (1964)	1. Neurological 2. To determine neurological status/integrity, to diagnose neurologic abnormality 3. Formal 4. Evaluation	Behavioral state, primitive reflexes, tone, posture, voluntary movement	Newborn 38–42 weeks' gestation

Psychometric Qualities	Clinical Implications	Source
Test-retest: .67–.83 Interrater reliability: .93–.97	Attempts to differentiate among normal, disorganized, and dysfunctional infants	Physical and Occupational Therapy in Pediatrics 5(4): 13, 1985
Test-retest reliability: .51–.85 Interrater reliability: .85 Age-related changes	Rather long to administer Requires a great deal of handling of the infant Incorporates state into testing procedures	Psychological Corp, PO Box 839954, San Antonio, TX 78283-3954
No reliability data Some descriptive information on predictive value	Used for both full term and preterm infants Quick and simple	Clinics in Developmental Medicine No. 79, J.B. Lippincott Co., Philadelphia, PA 19105
Interobserver reliability varies: behavioral state good, muscle tone poor Test-retest: .70–1.00 Sensitivity: .80	Lengthy exam Provides a great deal of descriptive information Application of "optimality" Stresses state control	Clinics in Developmental Medicine No. 63, J.B. Lippincott Co., Philadelphia, PA 19105

Table 2.3. continued

Name	1. Perspective 2. Purpose 3. Class 4. Category	Areas Assessed	Population
Nursing Child Assessment Satellite Training Teaching and Feeding Scales (NCAST), Barnard KE (1979)	1. Adaptive-transactive 2. To assess parental responsiveness to infant and the interaction of infant-caregiver 3. Informal 4. Assessment	Sensitivity to cues, response to distress, social-emotional growth, fostering cognitive growth, clarity of cues, responsiveness to parent	Teaching 0–3 years Feeding 0–1 year
Peabody Developmental Motor Scales, Folio M, Fewell R (1983)	1. Developmental 2. To determine developmental level 3. Formal 4. Evaluation	Reflexes, gross motor, fine motor	0–83 months
Pediatric Evaluation of Disability Inventory (PEDI), Haley SM, Coster WJ, Ludlow IH, Haltiwanger JT, Andrellos P (1992)	1. Functional 2. To determine functional deficits, monitor progress, and evaluate program 3. Formal 4. Assessment	Self-care, mobility, and social function	6 months–71/2 years
Quick Neurological Screening Test (QNST), Matti M, Sterling H, Spalding N (1978)	1. Neuromotor 2. To determine risk for learning disabilities 3. Formal 4. Screening	Motor maturity, fine and gross motor control, motor planning, spatial organization, visual and auditory perception, balance	6–17 years

Psychometric Qualities	Clinical Implications	Source
Discriminate validity: indicates differences between normal sample and infants born preterm, abused or FTT Predictive validity feeding: .72–.79 with HOME; teaching: .66 with PDI, .67 with MDI Percent agreement high	Provides information on interaction through structured situations that limit spontaneity	NCAST Publications, Seattle, WA
Test-retest reliability excellent Interrater reliability excellent Concurrent validity with BSID: .37–.36	Scoring allows crediting of emerging skills Activity cards available but of limited use	DLM Teaching Resources, One DLM Park, Allen, TX 75002
Standardized on 412 children Reliability > .90	Can be administered through structured interview Measures functional skill, capability and performance as indicated by caregiver assistance and environmental modifications	PEDI Research Group, Dept. of Rehab. Medicine, New England Medical Center Hospital, No. 75/750 Washington Street, Boston, MA 02111-1901
Test-retest reliability: .81 Interrater reliability: .93 Identify 70–73% of children with LD Correlation with Bender: .51, with WRAT: .50–.48	Indicates need for further psychoeducational evaluation	Western Psychological Services, 12031 Wilshire Blvd, Los Angeles, CA 90025

Table 2.3. continued

Name	1. Perspective 2. Purpose 3. Class 4. Category	Areas Assessed	Population
Scales of Independent Behavior (SIB), Bruininks RH, Woodcock RW, Wetherman RF, Hill BK (1984)	1. Developmental/ Functional 2. To determine level of independence across functional activities 3. Formal 4. Evaluation	Motor, social and communication, personal and community living, behavior problems	Birth–adult
Screening Test for Evaluating Preschoolers (First Step), Miller LJ (1993)	1. Developmental 2. To identify children in need of comprehensive evaluation 3. Formal 4. Screening	Cognition, communication, motor, social-emotional, adaptive	2 years, 9 months–6 years, 2 months
Sensory Integration and Praxis Test (SIPT), Ayres J (1989)	1. Sensory 2. To determine sensory processing abilities 3. Formal 4. Evaluation	Vestibular, proprioception, kinesthesia, tactile, visual	4 years–8 years, 11 months
Test of Infant Motor Performance (TIMP), Campbell SK, Girolami G, Kolobe T, Oston E, Lenke M (research edition: 1993)	1. Motor patterns 2. To identify deficits in postural control 3. Formal 4. Assessment	Ability to orient and stabilize head in space and response to stimulation, body alignment, selective control of distal movements, antigravity control of extremities	32 weeks' gestation–4 months post term

Psychometric Qualities	Clinical Implications	Source
Norm-referenced No reliability or validity provided	Some unique items relating motor skills with ability to perform functional activities Items related to program goals	DLM Teaching Resources, Allen, TX 75002
Internal consistency: .88–.91 Test-retest reliability: .93 Interrater reliability: .94	Strong psychometrics Games are fun, materials interesting Computer-assisted scoring format Requires specialized training and certification to administer	Psychological Corp, PO Box 39954, San Antonio, TX 78283-3954
Norm-referenced Multiple validity studies indicate test can be used to differentiate diagnostic groups, correlation with K-ABC, BOTMP among others Test-retest reliability: .31–.74 Interrater reliability: .51–.99 (most being above .90)	Not to be used with children with severe neuromotor dysfunction Recommend two testing sittings	Western Psychological Services, 12031 Wilshire Blvd, Los Angeles, CA 90025
Internal consistency: .98 Correlation with medical risk and age: .85	Attempts to capture postural control and response to movement rather than skill development In research version only No norms Minimal reliability and validity data	Suzanne Campbell, University of Illinois, Dept of Physical Therapy, 1919 W Taylor St, Chicago, IL 60612

Table 2.3. continued

Name	1. Perspective 2. Purpose 3. Class 4. Category	Areas Assessed	Population
Test of Sensory Functions in Infants (TSFI), DeGangi G, Greenspan S (1989)	1. Sensory 2. To measure sensory processing and reactivity 3. Formal 4. Assessment	Tactile deep pressure, visual-tactile integration, adaptive motor, ocular-motor, reactivity to vestibular stimulation	4–18 months
Toddler and Infant Motor Evaluation (TIME), Miller LJ (1994)	1. Motor performance 2. To assess repertoire of movement through observation 3. Informal 4. Assessment	Neurological foundations, stability, mobility, motor organization	Birth–42 months
Transdisciplinary Play Based Assessment, Linder T (1990)	1. Adaptive-transactive Developmental 2. To determine developmental skill level, learning style, and interaction through structured play 3. Informal 4. Assessment	Cognition, communication and language Sensorimotor, social-emotional	6 months–6 years

Psychometric Qualities	Clinical Implications	Source
Domain validity moderate-high Construct validity false normal rate of 75% Interobserver reliability high Best results at 7–18 months	May prove useful in predicting subtle SI dysfunction early	Western Psychological Services, 12031 Wilshire Blvd, Los Angeles, CA 90025
Pilot edition: interrater reliability > .90	Parent is only adult in contact with child Information gained through observation Attempts to gain information on quality of movement, quantity, and skill acquisition Requires a great deal of practice to record observations	Therapy Skill Builders, PO Box 42050, Tucson, AZ 85733
No reliability or validity data provided	Primarily observation Involves parents Links learning style with skill performance and problem-solving	Paul H. Brookes Publishing Co, PO Box 10624, Baltimore, MD 21285-0624

Neurological/Neuromotor

Items on a neurological exam are based on biological processes and the subsystems of the central nervous system: reflexes, tone, and automatic or postural reactions. They are used for screening, diagnosis, and prognosis of evident neurological disturbances and for evaluating changes in neurobehavioral organization over time.

Behavioral

Most are criterion-referenced instruments, used to obtain information on a variety of developmental areas. They are widely used in early intervention and school-based programs. Many instruments have accompanying curriculum and/or activity guides.

Sensory-Motor

These are used to obtain information on the child's perception of, processing of, and reactivity to primary sensory input (tactile, vestibular, proprioception, visual, and auditory).

Functional

These measurements are used to assess the performance of functional tasks and the degree of assistance needed to perform functional tasks (feeding, dressing, mobility, community independence) in determining level of impairments vs. limitations vs. disability vs. handicap.

Adaptive-Transactive

These instruments assess behavioral skills in conjunction with a dynamic interaction, most often with primary caregiver. They provide valuable information on behavioral styles and individual variations of the child.

Motor Performance

These are assessments of the quality of a motor activity and movement patterns.

CLINICAL OBSERVATIONS

Reflexes, Righting Reactions, Automatic Reactions

Primitive reflexes and the righting, automatic and equilibrium reactions should be assessed by criteria established by the authors of the neuromotor measurement instrument selected, for example, the NBAS for the full term neonate, the PDMS for infants and very young children, or the IMS for the preterm infant. The procedure developed by Fiorentino can also be used.

Range of Motion (ROM)

1. Children born full term (Table 2.4)
   a. Upper extremities: similar to adults, although elbow extension can be limited as much as 30° in the full term infant
   b. Lower extremities: substantial variation exists in reported measurements of lower extremity range of motion. There is a tendency for increased amount of flexion at birth for the child born full term because of neural(CNS maturation), mechanical (position), and environmental (interuterine crowding) factors. This flexor bias decreases over time
2. Children born preterm (Table 2.5)
   a. Lack of flexor bias that is seen at birth in infants born full term is due to lack of interuterine crowding, CNS immaturity, and extensor positioning
   b. Although extension bias decreases slightly over time, infants born preterm never demonstrate the extreme flexion that is seen in infants born full term
3. Considerations in accurately measuring joint ROM in infants and toddlers
   a. Lack of consensus regarding joint ROM values and methodology

Table 2.4. Average Value of Selected Lower Extremity Range of Motion, Birth through Five Years: Full-Term Infants

	Central Tendency Values and Range of Reported Values (reported in degrees)						
	Birth	6 wk	3 months	6 months	1 yr	3 yr	5 yr
Hip extension	34.2	19	7	7	7	7	7
Limitation							
Hip abduction	72.7						
In 90° flexion							
In extension	55.5				59.3	59.3	54.3
	(32–91)						
Hip adduction	6.4				30.5	30.5	23.8
Hip external rotation	91.9						
In flexion	(45–137)						
In extension	90	48	45	53.1	58	56	38.5
Hip internal rotation	64						
In flexion	(35–100)						
In extension	33	24	26	24	37.5	39	34
Knee extension	17.9				5.4	5.4	5.4
Limitation	(0–43.3)						
Popliteal angle	27		18	10.5	0		
	(20–40)		(15–30)	(5–15)	0		

Table 2.5. Average Value of Selected Joint Measurements: Preterm Infants (Ranges in Parentheses)

	Birth	4 months	8 months	12 months
Hip extension	166.6 (155–175)	161.4 (150–178)	163.1 (120–180)	164.1 (90–180)
Hip abduction (extension)	62.2 (50–90)	61.4 (40–90)	61.1 (35–90)	67.9 (15–90)
Popliteal angle	50.8 (125–180)	144.0 (112–180)	144.1 (117–180)	146 (125–175)
Angle dorsiflexion	127.5 (105–145)	127.7 (101–150)	122.9 (90–160)	118.5 (102–160)
Scarf sign	1.52 cm (0+4 cm)	–.08 cm (–5–+4 cm)	.27 cm (–4–+4 cm)	1.2 cm (1–2 cm)
Elbow extension	178.6 (165–180)	174.5 (160–180)	179.8 (175–180)	180
Wrist extension	98 (95–120)	103.7 (90–135)	100.2	101.2 (90–130)

b. Variation in reported reliability of goniometric measurements, possibly due to differences among goniometers (size, number system, and material)

c. Bony landmarks not fully developed and covered by increased fat in infants, making it difficult to palpate and line up the goniometer

d. Edema, pain, adhesions, strength deficits, and muscle hypertrophy can all affect accuracy of measurement

Muscle Tone

1. Describing tone
   a. Quantitative system
      - Flaccid
      - Decreased resistance to passive movement
      - Normal
      - Initial increase to passive movement and then relaxation to normal as movement continues
      - Consistent increase of tone throughout movement

   b. Descriptive system (Table 2.6)

   c. Distribution of tone: tone varies in relation to areas of the body or side of the body and may be different in relation to activities and position.

Muscle Testing

1. Manual Muscle Strength Test
   a. Infant:
      - Through observation
      - Limited to muscle groups
      - Focus on essential information
      - Observe for a symmetrical pattern of performance
      - Observe for compensating pattern
      - Grading system:
        x—present and strong
        o—absent
        T—trace, contraction palpated but no movement seen
   b. Children:
      - Consider body weight and size when consider level of resistance
      - Estimate through observation of muscle action in antigravity positions—arc of motion against gravity, i.e., assuming hands and knees position, bottom lifting, bringing feet to mouth
      - Observe for a symmetrical pattern of performance
      - Observe for compensatory movements
      - Isolated joint actions and specific muscle testing should be limited to children with language development appropriate to follow traditional MMT instructions. approximately 7–10 years of age

Muscle Power

1. Isometric power—ability to hold a position against gravity or known resistance. Apply force to muscle in shortened range
2. Isotonic power—ability of muscle to move through range with resistance applied throughout
3. Eccentric power—ability to resist a force as muscle is lengthened
4. Concentric power—ability to resist a force as muscle is shortened
5. Repetitive power—ability to produce adequate power for 10 repetitions
6. Speed of contraction—ability to adapt quickly throughout range

In young children and/or children with developmental disabilities, power can and should be assessed in functional developmental positions. For example, the squat-to-stand maneuver assesses eccentric control of the gastrocnemius and quadriceps muscle groups when the child moves down into the squat; when rising to a standing position, eccentric control of the hamstrings and concentric control of the quadriceps is assessed. At full upright, concentric control of gluteal muscle group is assessed. Repetitive power can be assessed by asking the child to repeat the squat-to-stand maneuver several times. Asking the child to start and stop at different speeds will assess the speed of contraction.

Table 2.6. Muscle Tone: Descriptive System

Hypotonia			Normal
Severe	Moderate	Mild	
Active			
Inability to resist gravity, lack of cocontraction at proximal joints, limited voluntary movements	Decreased tone primarily in axial muscles and proximal muscles of the extremities, interferes with length of time a posture can be sustained	Decreased tone interferes with axial muscle cocontractions, delays initiation of movement	Quick and immediate postural adjustment during movement, ability to use muscles in synergic and reciprocal patterns for stability and mobility depending on task
Passive			
Joint hyperextensibility, no resistance to movement imposed by examiner, full or excessive passive ROM	Mild resistance to movement when imposed by examiner in distal parts of extremities only; elbow and knee joint hyperextensibility	Mild resistance in proximal as well as distal segments, full ROM	Body parts resist displacement, momentarily maintain new posture when placed in space, and can rapidly follow changing movements imposed by examiner

Isokinetic

1. Follow instructions provided by manufacturers
2. Minimal amount of normative data available
3. Effects of age, height, and weight must be taken into consideration

Posture

1. Axial region
   a. Torticollis
      - Observe the infant for asymmetry in supine, prone, and sitting. Typically, infants with torticollis will laterally flex head to the right and rotate the face and chin to the left

Hypertonia			Intermittent Tone
Mild	Moderate	Severe	
Delay in postural adjustment, poor coordination, slowness of movement	Limits speed, coordination, variety of movement patterns, and active ROM	Severe stiffness of muscles in stereotypic patterns, limits active ROM, little or no ability to move against gravity, very limited patterns of movement	Occasional and unpredictable resistance to postural changes alternating with normal adjustment; may have difficulty initiating active movement or sustaining posture
Resistance to change of posture in part of or throughout the range, poor ability to accommodate to passive movements	Resistance to change of posture throughout the range, limited passive ROM at some joints	ROM limited, unable to overcome resistance of muscle to complete full range	Unpredictable resistance to imposed movements alternating with complete absence of resistance

- Assess passive and active range of motion of the neck and upper extremities to determine whether limitations and/or contractures are present
- Assess motor development in order to determine influence of torticollis on developmental milestone acquisition

b. Scoliosis
- A minimal amount of clothing should be worn by the child
- Align the child with a plumb line (physical or imaginary)
- The child should assume a natural standing posture with feet together
- Observe the position of the head, the trunk, the hips, and the legs from the front, back, and side noting any asymmetries
  - Unequal shoulder level
  - Scapular prominence
  - Uneven waist lines/hip prominence
  - Pelvic asymmetry

- Unequal distance between arms and body
- Unequal knee level
- Forward bending test
    - Sit or kneel behind the child with your eyes level to the waist
    - Ask the child to bend forward from the waist until spine is approximately parallel to the floor, knees are straight, and arms are hanging with palms together
    - Observe for compensatory unilateral rib hump
- From the side
    - Note excessive thoracic kyphosis or excessive lumbar lordosis
- Assess flexibility of the hip: Thomas test
- MMT
- Inquire about functional limitations and/or pain during participation in sports, dancing, or other activities

Disorders of the Hip

1. Congenital dislocation of the hip (Fig. 2.2)
    a. Physical inspection
        - Ortolani: examines hip reducibility (return dislocated femoral head back into acetabulum)
            - Infant supine
            - Hip and knees in 90° of flexion
            - Grasp thigh with middle finger over greater trochanter and thumb on medial thigh
            - Other hand stabilizes pelvis
            - Gently lift the thigh to align femoral head and acetabulum and abduct the hip to slide the head over the acetabular rim into the socket
            - Examiner will feel a definite "clunk"

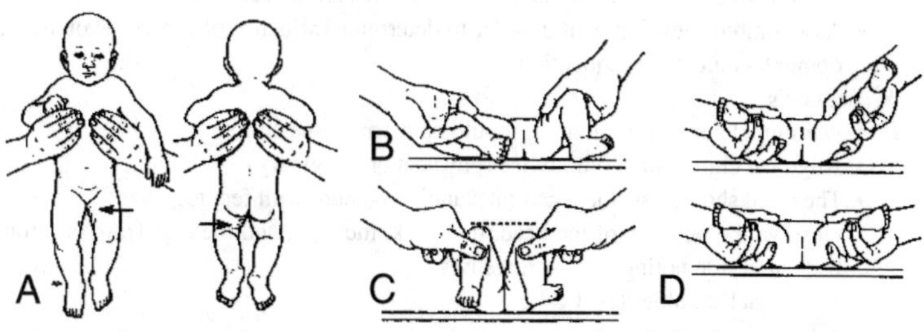

Figure 2.2. Signs of hip dislocation. **A.** Asymmetrical skin folds. **B.** Limited abduction. **C.** Apparent shortening of one thigh. **D.** Examination to elicit relocation or dislocation.

- Barlow: examines the ability of the hip to dislocate
  - Infant supine
  - Knees and hips flexed at 90°
  - Grasp the thigh with thumb medially over the lesser trochanter
  - Other hand stabilizes pelvis
  - Apply gentle downward pressure while abducting the hip
  - As femoral head slips over acetabulum rim a subtle "clunk" is felt

Sensory Testing

1. Infants: used to determine intact sensation. Apply noxious stimuli (i.e., pin prick) when infant is drowsy and observe for withdrawal, crying, or grimacing. Proceed distal to proximal. Flexor withdrawal response is indicative of spinal cord level response; crying, grimacing and/or startle responses can help determine level of intact sensation.
2. Children with head trauma: child's response to specific sensory stimuli changes as level of consciousness changes. Stimuli through intact auditory, visual, olfactory, gustatory, and pain pathways evoke a response at all levels of consciousness except V.
   - Level IV: generalized response to any stimuli; response is same regardless of stimuli
   - Level III: individualized response to specific stimuli; delay often occurs prior to response (Table 2.7)
   - Level II: specific testing of proprioception; sharp-dull and 2-point discrimination limited by child's cognition and age

Table 2.7. Localized Response to Sensory Stimuli—Level III

Sensory Tract	Stimulus Examples	Response
Auditory	Voice Bell Hand clapping	Eye opening Looking toward stimulus Turning head toward/away from stimulus
Visual	Threat near eyes Bright object Familiar toy Familiar person	Blinking Focusing and tracking
Olfactory	Ammonia	Grimace or turn away
Gustatory	Sugar Lemon	Smile Grimace
Pain	Squeeze muscle belly Squeeze nail bed, pin prick	Pull extremity away Look toward pain

BALANCE

There are clinical tools that can be utilized in addition to static balance and dynamic balance tasks assessed on standardized measurement batteries.

Clinical Test for Sensory Interaction and Balance (CTSIB)

1. Assessment of Standing Balance
   Individual postural sway while standing for a maximum period of 30 seconds is observed in each of six conditions (Fig. 2.3)
2. Scoring:
   - Numeric ranking system based on amount of sway
     1 = minimal
     2 = mild
     3 = moderate
     4 = fall
   - Record amount of time the individual maintains erect standing with a stopwatch
   - Record body displacement from grid or plumb line
   - Record changes in perception (dizziness, nausea) and movement strategies used to maintain stability
3. Interpretation:
   a. Most children over 9 years of age easily maintain stability under all conditions
   b. Abnormal reliance on vision or increase in sway under conditions 3–6 indicates sensory interaction deficit

Functional Reach

1. Procedure
   a. Child must be able to stand for at least one minute without any type of assistance
   b. Allow two practice trials and perform five test trials
   c. Place yardstick at acromion process
   d. Hold dominant arm out
   e. Make a fist
   f. Measure at head of 3rd metacarpal
   g. Ask child to reach as far forward as possible without taking a step
   h. Measure distance reached (Table 2.8).
2. Interpretation: Reach scores below critical values (–2 SD) may indicate a delay

ORAL-MOTOR AND FEEDING

Facial and Intraoral Anatomy

1. Observation: deformity or asymmetry
2. Palpation: tongue, jaw, palate
3. Radiographic

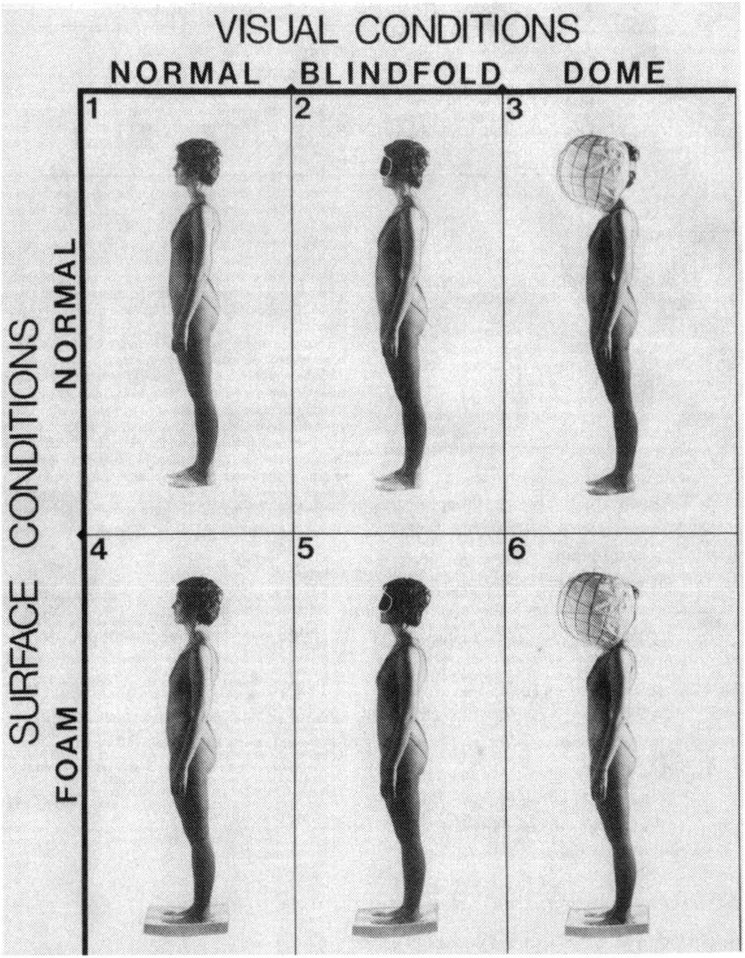

Figure 2.3. Sequence of six conditions for testing the influence of sensory interaction on balance.

Table 2.8. Functional Reach Scores Ages 5–15

Age	Mean Reach (cm)	Critical Reach (cm)
5–6	21.17	16.79
7–8	24.21	20.57
9–10	27.97	25.56
11–12	32.79	29.68
13–15	32.30	29.58

Oral Function

1. Rooting reaction
2. Gag reflex
3. Bite reaction

Suck—Swallow

1. Suck
   a. Negative: suction created within oral cavity
   b. Positive: expression consisting of stripping the milk from the nipple
   c. Characterized by bursts (group of sucks less than 1 second interspersed with pauses)
   d. Non-nutritive: shorter bursts
      - hand-to-mouth
      - sucking on pacifier
      - nipple over finger and insert in mouth with slight downward pressure on the tongue note lowering and elevation of mandible and acceptance of nipple
   e. Nutritive
      - Higher rate of swallowing
      - Offer nipple: note mouth opening, lip closure (lips should purse around nipple), rhythmicity of sucking and frequency of gasping, gagging, and/or choking
   f. Strength of suck
      - Attempt to pull nipple out of mouth
      - Infants seal should tighten and head will come forward
   g. Endurance: 15-30 minutes

Behavioral: observe child feeding and note the following:

1. Spoon (try various textures and tastes)
   a. Mouth quiet until food presented?
   b. Graded mouth opening to receive spoon?
   c. Good lip closure around spoon?
   d. Food cleaned from spoon with upper lip?
   e. Stable position of head maintained?

   f. Effective mobility of tongue and jaw?
   g. Swallow and breathing coordinated?
2. Drinking out of a cup
   a. Jaw excursion graded?
   b. Jaw sufficiently stabilized to allow normal placement of cup?
   c. Lip closure adequate?
   d. Coordination of drinking, breathing, and swallowing?
3. Biting and chewing
   a. Jaw movement: early up and down "munching" or more mature rotary movement?
   b. Tongue moving laterally to keep food between teeth?
   c. Lips closed adequately?
4. Self-feeding
5. Associated behaviors
   a. Frequent gagging or choking?
   b. Vomiting (when and how often?)
   c. Drooling
   d. Attitude toward feeding: relaxed? tight? interactive?
   e. Expression of food preferences: texture? avoidance? flavor?

Assessment Scales (Table 2.3)

1. Pre-speech Assessment Scale (PSAS)
   a. Birth through two years
   b. Twenty-seven pre-speech performance areas divided into 6 categories
2. Oral-Motor Feeding Rating Scale
   a. 1–3 years of age
   b. Five sections
      - Identifying information
      - Oral-motor/feeding patterns
      - Related areas of function
      - Respiration-phonation
      - Rating scale synopsis
3. Neonatal Oral-Motor Assessment Scale (NOMAS)
   a. Neonate
   b. Evaluates jaw and tongue movements in nutritive and non-nutritive sucking modes
4. Behavioral Assessment Scale of Oral Function in Feeding; most useful for infants > 8 months

BIOMECHANICAL ANALYSIS

Kinematics

1. Descriptive analysis of a movement pattern via joint or segment position, joint angles, time, displacement (linear, angular) velocities, and accelerations

2. Imaging techniques: highly sophisticated motion analysis systems are available, generally in motor control laboratories or gait analysis laboratories. Three types are available (Table 2.9):
   a. Cinematography
   b. Videography
   c. Optolectric system

Kinetics:
represents the pattern of forces that underlie movement

Electromyography:
describes electrical activity of a muscle
interpretation requires corresponding movement analysis

Table 2.9. Advantages and Disadvantages of Kinematic Systems

Consideration	Cinematography	Videography	Optoelectric
Ease of use	Somewhat sophisticated	Sophisticated	Very sophisticated
Cost	Moderate to high, except cost of conversion equipment	Moderate, except cost of conversion equipment	Expensive
Frequency	>= 64 Hz	60 Hz (U.S.A.) < 50 Hz (Europe)	>= 64 Hz
Encumbrance to movement	Minimal	Minimal	Some
Time to attach	Minimal	Minimal	Moderate
Availability of data for analysis	Film processing and conversion of data high	Instant replay; has capability for instant conversion	Instant conversion
Lighting	Extra lighting required indoors	No extra lighting required for 2D, but may be useful; required for 3D	Extra lighting required
Visual record	Available	Available	Not available unless coupled with video
Laboratory vs. naturalistic setting	Both	Both	Laboratory

SOFT SIGNS

Assessment of soft signs emphasizes how they may affect a child's functional performance on tasks involving movement, perception, and spatial organization.

Many of the items examined under soft signs are incorporated into formal (standardized or criterion-referenced) instruments previously described.

Developmental soft signs:

imply a state of immature neurological function

1. Awkwardness
2. Motor overflow
3. Right-left confusion
4. Mild oculomotor difficulties

Neurological soft signs:

abnormalities that do not occur at any time during development

1. Persistence of primitive reflexes
2. Reflex asymmetries

Postural control

1. Muscle tone
2. Primitive postural reflexes: primitive reflexes may be observed in positions of stress until 8 or 9 years of age
   a. Hands and knees position to test ATNR, STNR
   b. Schilder's arm extension test
   c. ATNR sunshine position
   d. Purdue reflex test
3. Vestibular function and equilibrium
   a. Postrotary nystagmus test
   b. Prone extension position
   c. Romberg position
   d. Mann's position
   e. Floor ataxia test
4. Fine motor movements
   a. Diadokinesis
   b. Thumb-to-finger touching
   c. Ability to cross midline
5. Eye-hand coordination

PULMONARY FUNCTION

Pulmonary Function Tests

1. Forced vital capacity (FVC)
2. Forced expiratory volume in 1 second (FEV_1)
3. Ratio of FEV to FVC (FEV/FVC)
4. Forced expiratory flow (FEF_{25-75})
5. Peak expiratory flow rate (PEFR)
6. Residual volume (RV)
7. Functional residual capacity (FRC)

Clinical Observations

1. History
2. Chest
   a. Unmoving—shape and symmetry of the thorax; observe for pectus excavatum, funnel chest pectus carinatum, and scoliosis
   b. Moving—respiratory rate, symmetry: compare right and left thorax
   c. Synchrony—compare thoracic and abdominal movement
   d. Retractions—indrawing of thorax during inspiration
   e. General appearance—skeletal abnormalities
3. Head and neck
   a. Flaring of the nose
   b. Head bobbing
   c. Audible sounds—expiratory grunting
   d. Color
      - Cyanosis
      - Pallor
      - Plethora
4. Coughing and Sneezing; stimulate oral or nasal pharynx to elicit cough or sneeze to determine whether functional
5. Auscultation; breath sounds
   a. Normal—rustle, reach maximum intensity during inspiration
   b. Bronchial—harsh and loud heard throughout inspiration and expiration
   c. Decreased—less intense than normal
   d. Abnormal sounds
   e. Crackles/rales
   f. Wheezes/rhonchi
   g. Extrapulmonary sounds
   h. Rubs

6. Palpation
7. Percussion
   a. Not particularly accurate or helpful in neonate unless therapist is experienced
   b. Used to identify abnormally dense lung and diaphragmatic motion in older children

Strength, posture, flexibility, and endurance should also be measured in older children and adolescents

Vital signs (Tables 2.10 and 2.11)

PRESEASON SCREENING EVALUATION OF ADOLESCENT ATHLETES

Components

1. Muscle strength
2. Power
3. Endurance
4. Speed
5. Agility
6. Flexibility
7. Cardiovascular endurance
8. Joint Stability
9. Posture

Table 2.10. Normal Heart Rates and Blood Pressures for Children

	Birth–1 month	Up to 3 Years	>3 Years
Heart rate (bpm)	120–200	100–180	70–150
Blood pressure (mm HG)			
Systolic	60–90	75–130	90–140
Diastolic	30–60	45–90	50–80

Table 2.11. Normal Respiratory Rates for Children

Age	Breaths per Minute
Birth–1 month	35–55
Up to 6 years	20–30
6–10 years	15–25
10–16 years	12–20

Contraindications (Table 2.12)

Physical Fitness Test Battery

Physical Best: The AAHPERD Guide to Physical Fitness, Education and Assessment. Reston, VA: The American Alliance for Health, Physical Education, Recreation and Dance; 1989: focuses on health related fitness: aerobic endurance, body composition, flexibility, muscular strength, muscular endurance

ARENA ASSESSMENT

This involves simultaneous assessment of a child by various disciplines. A team designs a scheme prior to assessment so that a common sample of behaviors can be observed. It is primarily used for program planning of a child identified as having a developmental disability or delay.

Purpose

1. Obtain a holistic, integrated view of the child
2. Determine the interrelationships across domains
3. Reduce multiple handling of infant and child

Table 2.12. Contraindications for Exercise Testing in Pediatric Patients

1. Acute febrile condition
2. Acute inflammatory cardiac disease, e.g., pericarditis, myocarditis, acute rheumatic heart disease
3. Congestive heart failure—uncontrolled
4. Asthmatic child who is dyspneic at rest, or whose FEV or PEF are less than 60% of height
5. Acute renal disease
6. Acute hepatitis, during 3 months' onset
7. Insulin-dependent diabetic who did not take his prescribed insulin or who is ketoacidotic
8. Drug overdose affecting cardiorespiratory response to exercise, e.g., digitalis or quinidine toxicity, salicylism, or antidepressants

Components

1. Team—full range of team members. Members should be chosen from the predetermined and/or desired outcomes. Members must be confident and have ability to share information and techniques
2. Facilitator—one person with child

Process

1. No script—child and family driven
2. Sequence should be naturalistic in response to child; examples: greeting—tasks—snack—separation and reunion—storytime—free play—exit
3. This sequence should obtain information in the:
   a. Physical/motor domain
   b. Psychoeducational domain
   c. Psychosocial domain

Staffing

1. Parents may or may not be present
2. Time needed to analyze and synthesize assessment findings, not simply relate development levels and judge status of child

Outcome

1. Historical portrait of intervention
2. Qualitative and quantitative descriptions of the child
3. Identification of critical areas of strengths and needs
4. Developmental picture

Advantages

1. Gives thorough picture of child
2. Is process driven
3. Can be geared to existing outcomes, goals, and objectives

Disadvantages

1. Time-consuming
2. Requires a highly skilled facilitator and skilled team members

APPROACHES TO ASSESSMENT

Bottom-up Approach (Figure 2.4)

1. Traditional deficit-driven model to assessment
2. Professional assesses child, determines strengths, needs, and deficit areas; professional determines goals based on findings and determines intervention strategies
3. Traditionally used for identification of disability or delay and/or during diagnostic process

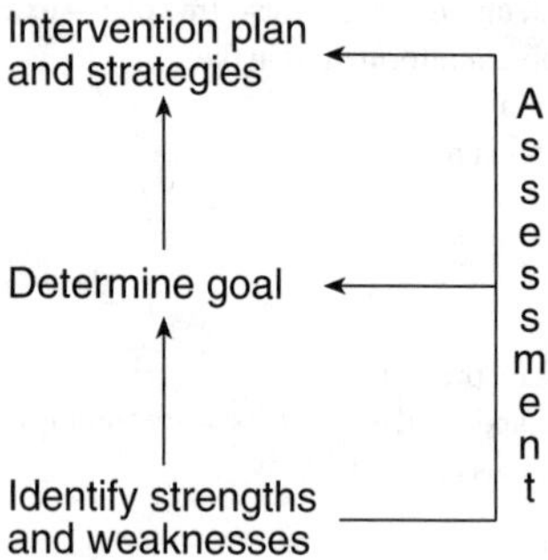

Figure 2.4. Bottom-up approach.

Top-Down Approach (Fig. 2.5)

1. Outcome-driven model to assessment
2. Desired outcomes determined first; identify obstacles and strengths of the child and family to obtain outcome; identify strategies to improve performance, bypass obstacles, and reach desired outcome
3. Ongoing assessment takes place at any point, i.e., identifying obstacles, identifying strengths, and adapting intervention strategies
4. Primarily used for program planning

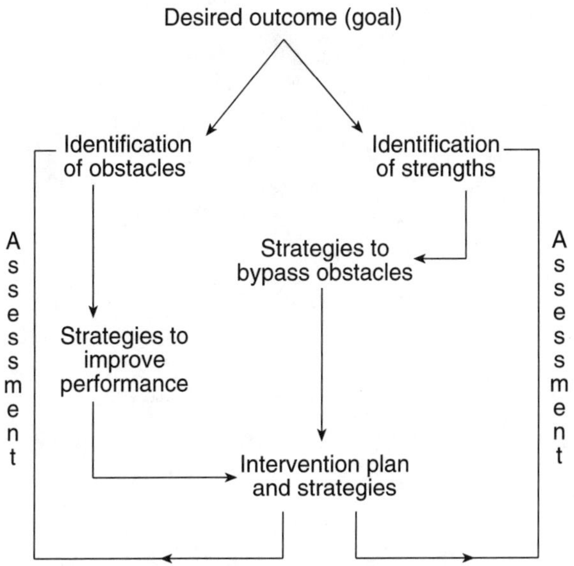

Figure 2.5. Top-down approach.

3 / Pediatric Disorders

Holly Lea Cintas

The spectrum of pediatric disorders encountered by physical therapists and related professionals is quite broad, and a child's diagnosis may encompass several body systems. For these reasons, pediatric disorders discussed in this chapter are listed alphabetically, rather than by system or age. Assessment information is included only in those instances when an assessment exists for a specific disorder. Otherwise, comprehensive information on assessment is included in Chapter 2: Measurement.

CLASSIFICATIONS

In an effort to describe children beyond their clinical diagnoses, signs, and symptoms, a standardized classification was used for the description of pediatric disorders. The World Health Organization (WHO) ICIDH classification discussed below could be used for this purpose; however, Nagi's classification may have some advantages over the ICIDH classification, principally its avoidance of the term "handicap." For this and other reasons noted below, Nagi's classification scheme is used for this chapter.

WHO International Classification of Impairment, Disability and Handicap (ICIDH)

1. Developed by Wood in 1980
2. Conceptualizes disablement as a continuum proceeding from disease to impairment to disability to handicap
3. Focuses on functional ability rather than comparison to normalcy
4. Provides categories for patient problems as well as means for documenting areas in which problems do not exist so that an individual can be described comprehensively
5. Digit-coding system is used to classify each problem as present or absent; additional, individualized categories may be added
6. Specific conditions can be described or analyzed on several levels, according to a hierarchy:
   a. **Disorder or pathology: first level** of dysfunction: disease or injury to tissues, organs, or systems as identified by care providers and/or diagnostic testing
   b. **Impairment: second level:** external manifestation of a disorder; signs and symptoms of the condition; typically described using physical therapy assessments of strength and range of motion
   c. **Disability: third level:** restriction of ability of a person in relation to his or her immediate environment as a result of an impairment; includes communication, per-

sonal care activities, posture, locomotion, and manipulation; level at which an individual's impairment is reflected in goal-directed behaviors incorporating environmental interaction

d. **Handicap: fourth level:** classification of circumstances which prevent an individual from realizing his or her full potential in society due to the presence of an impairment or disability; described in terms of personal, family, and societal limitations on the individual with respect to employment, education, family roles, leisure activities, financial independence, and social integration

Nagi's System of Classification (Nagi, 1991)

1. Substitutes "functional limitations" for **ICIDH's** disability
2. Substitutes disability for "handicap"; "handicap" may be viewed as a derogatory term in the United States
3. Removes **ICIDH** linkage between impairment and disability; impairments may be multiple and may exist without disability
4. Accommodates levels of ability demonstrated by children more readily than **ICIDH**
5. Unlike **ICIDH,** does not use digital codes for clinical reporting purposes

PEDIATRIC DISORDERS DESCRIBED ACCORDING TO THE NAGI CLASSIFICATION[1]

Acquired Immune Deficiency Syndrome (AIDS)

1. **Pathology:**
   a. Viral infection which suppresses immune system function, principally through T-cell involvement; **AIDS** is the most severe manifestation of human immunodeficiency viral **(HIV)** infection
   b. Leads to the development of opportunistic infections
   c. Transmission secondary to maternal infection prenatally or perinatally or through breast milk, through introduction into the body of infected blood or blood products, by intravenous injection with contaminated needles, or by sexual contact with infected individuals without barrier protection
   d. HIV incubation stage may extend several years before development of AIDS; is typically shorter in infants and children than in adults

[1]The Disability Category has been excluded because it is highly variable depending on the cultural and social environment of an individual. In certain cases, the Pathology Category has been excluded when an impairment exists independent of pathology.

2. **Impairment:**
   a. **AIDS-related complex (ARC)** is a prodromal stage with all the characteristics of AIDS except opportunistic infections: includes low birth weight, failure-to-thrive, interstitial pneumonitis, chronic diarrhea, recurrent bacterial and viral infections including meningitis, additional multiple system problems and subsequent muscle weakness, and reduced opportunity for mobility
   b. **AIDS** includes all of above, often to a more severe degree, in addition to opportunistic infections such as cytomegalovirus (**CMV**), pneumocystis pneumonia, and disseminated candida infection
3. **Functional Limitations:**
   a. Proportional to the stage of the disease and associated symptoms
   b. Range from no apparent age-appropriate limitations to full loss of independent mobility
   c. Maternal illness and premature death may also result in limited functional and social opportunities
4. **Treatment Goals and Interventions:**
   a. **Goal:** Provide optimal quality of life experiences for the child through effective teamwork with all caregivers, especially family
      - Utilize treatment sessions as teaching sessions as appropriate
      - Select or fabricate equipment or assistive devices following in-depth consultation with all parties involved in the care of the child
      - Respect child, family, and other caregivers' needs in making determinations about level of care
      - Acknowledge the role of emotional support that can be provided by the physical therapist in addition to the physical aspects of caregiving
   b. **Goal:** Provide physical therapy interventions appropriate to child's age, level of function, severity of symptoms, and interests
      - Utilize developmental activities to promote mobility and increase child's functional capability whenever possible
      - Choose isolated joint exercises in instances where child cannot participate in higher level functional activities
      - Incorporate fine motor, social, and cognitive activities with gross motor activities
      - Use medium of play to accomplish physical therapy objectives
      - Communicate with physical therapists and caregivers who are or will be providing care in other settings to ensure smooth, planned transitions
5. **Supplemental Treatment:**
   a. Essential to minimize impact of the viral infection
   b. Medical care using drugs such as **AZT** and **DDI** is showing promise; however, prevention through education is currently the most effective approach in the treatment of AIDS and HIV

Amputations and Limb Deficiencies Specific to Children

1. **Pathology:**
   a. Congenital amputations or limb deficiencies are typically the result of limb maldevelopment occurring during the sensitive period of 4–7 weeks of gestational age
   b. Maternal thalidomide ingestion early in the sensitive period has been correlated with **amelia,** complete absence of a limb
   c. Partial absence of a limb, **meromelia,** has been identified in conjunction with thalidomide ingestion late in the critical period
   d. Amputation or limb deficits can also result from premature amnion rupture and subsequent band constriction around a portion of a limb, interrupting vascular supply and preventing continued vitality of that portion of the arm or leg
   e. Genetic disorders have been associated with some limb deficits such as polydactyly and ectrodactyly
2. **Impairment:**

Acheiria: absence of a hand

Amelia or Ectromelia: complete absence of a limb

Apodia: absence of a foot

Ectrodactyly: partial or complete absence of a digit; also refers to cleft hand or cleft foot, in which two or more digits are fused, leaving a central opening

Hemimelia or Meromelia: absence of some portion of a limb; refers to mild or moderate limb defects

Intercalary limb deficit: only the middle part of the limb is affected; proximal and distal portions are unaffected

Phocomelia: top portion of the limb is absent and the terminal part of the limb is attached higher than would normally be expected, for example, the hand may be attached to the shoulder

Polydactyly: extra digits are present on the hand or foot

Proximal Focal Femoral Deficiency: partial form of phocomelia in which the shaft of the femur is always short, the femoral head may not be present, or there may be no bony connection between the femoral head and shaft

Syndactyly: digits are fused together

Terminal limb deficit: unaffected parts do not exist below the affected portion of the limb

3. **Functional Limitations:**
   a. Dependent on the type and severity of the limb deficit
   b. In general, amputations treated with prostheses which support attainment of age-appropriate activities of daily living are not considered disabling
4. **Treatment Goals and Interventions:**
   a. **Goal:** Effective teamwork with child, family, and multiple health and educational providers
      - Consensus decisions are critical for timing of the introduction of a prosthesis, orthosis, or surgery

- Articulation of medical and educational interventions is necessary to address the child's developmental and musculoskeletal needs
- Child's temperament and response to interventions should be carefully monitored to increase the likelihood of prosthetic acceptance
- Environmental limitations on prosthetic use should be anticipated and discussed with the family; for example, can the child swim with it on?

b. **Goal:** Optimal achievement with upper extremity prosthetic use
- Infant may be fitted with 1st UE prosthesis when (s)he attains independent sitting, although earlier fitting may facilitate quadrupedal activity
- 2 years is optimal time to begin formal training for children with UE amputations
- Training strategies depend on choice of control systems (body powered or myoelectric), type of terminal device (hook, CAPP or hand), and client age and preference
  - Body-powered prostheses with hook terminal devices are lighter weight and relatively maintenance free
  - Myoelectric systems with hands are cosmetically more acceptable and permit more freedom of movement in the absence of a harness, but require frequent maintenance
- Motions utilized to open the terminal device for body powered prostheses:
  - Below elbow: humeral flexion
  - Above elbow: humeral flexion and scapular abduction
  - Shoulder disarticulation: biscapular abduction and chest expansion

c. **Goal:** Optimal achievement with lower extremity prosthetic use
- Prosthesis typically introduced when child pulls to stand, although earlier introduction preferred by some to promote quadrupedal function
- Prosthetic knee joint introduced at 3 years of age; adult type prosthesis at 5–6 years of age for most children with above knee amputations
- Training strategies are similar to those used for adults with age-appropriate pediatric adaptations
- Once consistent heel-strike is achieved, children respond well to treadmill training for improved neuromotor skill and cardiopulmonary endurance

5. **Supplemental Interventions:**

a. **Surgery** is frequently indicated to improve cosmesis and/or functional ability
- **Improved digitization** may be the outcome of separating fused digits or removing supranumerary digits, although this does not always result in functional improvement
- **Amputation** to remove nonfunctional tissue often results in improved prosthetic fitting and function; for example, **Symes amputation** may be done in a skeletally mature individual where distal flare of tibia and fibula are trimmed, whereas **ankle disarticulation** may be appropriate for an immature patient

b. **Biofeedback (auditory or visual)** may be useful for gait training to promote increased prosthetic weightbearing or stride length, and for training upper extremity movement strategies

Arthrogryposis Multiplex Congenita: see Multiple Congenital Contractures

Brachial Plexus Injury

1. **Pathology**:
   a. Compression or traction injury to the brachial plexus, typically unilateral
   b. May occur secondary to trauma to the shoulder from prenatal or postnatal events or anomalies such as cervical rib or abnormal thoracic vertebrae
   c. Most commonly associated with a difficult birth process, although compression by a car safety seat during a cross-country trip has been described
   d. Symptoms can range from swelling of the neural sheath to total avulsion of the nerve roots from the spinal cord, resulting in the interruption of sensory and/or motor impulse transmission
   e. Electromyography is useful in determining extent of nerve damage; prognosis is related to severity of injury rather than extent of involvement and is favorable in most instances
   f. Fractures of the clavicle or humerus, shoulder dislocation, and facial or phrenic nerve damage may co-exist
2. **Impairment:**

Sensory impairment is typically present; however, it may not correspond to motor involvement and is difficult to assess in infants. Although influenced by motor ability, the child's response to pin prick can be useful to determine baseline loss and recovery of function. Since denervated skin does not wrinkle in water, the presence of wrinkles after the "wrinkle test," immersion in water for 30 minutes at 40°C, may be used to monitor sensory recovery.

Motor impairment is analyzed by observation of spontaneous or elicited movements, muscle testing, and electromyography. It is categorized as follows:

a. **Erb's Palsy:** Upper plexus injury to C5 and C6 nerve roots may result in weakness or paralysis in the levator scapulae, rhomboids, deltoid, serratus anterior, supraspinatus, infraspinatus, biceps brachii, brachialis, brachioradialis, forearm supinator, and forearm extensors of the wrist, fingers, and thumb
b. **Klumpke Paralysis/Palsy:** Lower plexus injury to C7, C8, and T1 may result in distal weakness or paralysis in the wrist and finger flexors and extensors, and the intrinsic muscles in the hand
c. **Erb-Klumpke Paralysis/Palsy:** Mixed involvement which may include some or all

roots from C5 to T1; muscle weakness or paralysis dependent on which roots are included

3. **Functional Limitations:**
   a. Dependent on the severity and extent of sensory and motor impairment in the involved arm and the presence of associated conditions
   b. Infants may recover from traction injuries spontaneously, whereas recovery from avulsion injuries may be limited; if resolution does not occur within 4 months, prognosis for full recovery is unlikely
   c. Shoulder subluxation and contractures may develop secondary to muscle imbalance according to the following general pattern: glenohumeral adduction and internal rotation, elbow extension, forearm pronation, wrist and finger flexion
4. **Goals and Interventions**
   a. **Goal:** Avoid further damage
      - Early postnatal positioning in adduction, internal rotation, and supination may be utilized to limit further damage
      - 2-week recovery period suggested without active intervention except gentle range of motion
   b. **Goal:** Minimize or avoid contractures
      - Maintain range of motion through active and gentle passive exercise of the shoulder girdle, arm, and hand
      - Scapulo-humeral mobility is critical, but damage to the glenohumeral joint can occur if the humerus is mobilized more than 30° with the scapula manually held
      - Splinting of elbow, wrist, or hand may be indicated; splinting of shoulder is controversial
   c. **Goal:** Elicit active muscle function
      - Age-appropriate developmental activities
      - Dynamic weightbearing or loading of the extremity
      - Neuromuscular electrical stimulation may be considered
      - Temporary restriction of the uninvolved arm during therapy sessions may promote increased use of the affected arm
      - Goal-oriented sensorimotor activities with measurable behavioral outcomes are recommended
5. **Supplemental Interventions:**
   a. Surgical nerve repair or nerve reconstruction in infants with no recovery of the biceps or deltoid by 3 months of age
   b. Tendon transplantation or connective tissue elongation in older children

Brachycephaly (see Table 3.1)

Blount Disease (see Table 3.1)

Table 3.1. Joint Deformations in Infants and Children

Name or Location	Pathology or Contributing Factors	Impairment; Associated Factors	Treatment
Foot			
Calcaneovalgus	Prolonged breech position; uterine position forces foot into extreme dorsiflexion against lower leg; common in firstborns and females	Hyperdorsiflexed foot, often with valgus; high association with hip dislocation	Usually resolves without treatment, but taping may be necessary
Cavus Foot (Pes Cavus)	Muscle imbalance often associated with peroneal muscular atrophy, spina bifida, and poliomyelitis	Abnormally high medial and lateral longitudinal arches accompanied by flexed toes and calcaneovarus or valgus	Maintain joint mobility through exercise, especially length of toe flexors; maintain stability through orthotic support
Equinovarus (clubfoot):	Fetal confinement or fetal akinesia syndrome	Serious whole foot adduction problem, often associated with plantar flexion	Almost always requires surgical repair; good outcome if isolated problem, less positive if associated with additional problems
Equinus Foot (Pes Equinus)	Imbalance of muscle pull; leg length discrepancy; positional in flaccid paralysis; absence of weightbearing to maintain tendon length	Chronic calcaneal elevation usually due to shortening of the Tendo-achilles; high association with hamstring shortening, especially during standing and walking	Identify contributing factors, particularly role of hamstring and gastroc-soleus spasticity; utilize back stepping and sit-to-stand maneuvers to interrupt spastic pattern, exercises to elongate and activate; bracing, especially articulated MAFO

Table 3.1. continued

Name or Location	Pathology or Contributing Factors	Impairment; Associated Factors	Treatment
Metatarsus Adductus (Metatarsus Varus)	Compression of forefoot when legs flexed across the body during late gestation	Excessive adduction of forefoot; differentiated from equinovarus by hindfoot neutral or valgus position	Responds to manual stretching and avoidance of sleeping positions that sustain it; taping or casting may be necessary
Knee			
Genu Recurvatum	Congenital: fetal positioning and confinement, especially breech position; Musculoskeletal: joint laxity at the knee or imbalance in muscle strength or activation	Posterior tibial glide relative to femur is excessive, especially during standing and walking	Congenital: usually resolves without treatment except for positioning; Musculoskeletal: determination of cause (hypotonia, muscle imbalance) is critical to identify appropriate intervention
Genu Valgus	Medial knee instability, collapsed medial foot, muscle imbalance, degenerative joint disease	Tibia positioned laterally relative to femur; high association with coxa vara	Ankle orthosis can improve foot and knee alignment; monitor alignment during growth with joint disease
Genu Varus; Tibia Vara or Blount Disease	Lateral knee instability, medial growth disturbance of proximal tibial epiphysis	Lateral bowing of the tibia, often associated with obesity and early walking	May be progressive in spite of intervention; orthotic efforts first, then surgery

Table 3.1. continued

Name or Location	Pathology or Contributing Factors	Impairment; Associated Factors	Treatment
Tibial Torsion (exaggerated)	Congenital: rotatory forces placed on knee joint and lower leg during gestational compression	Excessive rotation of tibia relative to femur, spiraling of tibial shaft; almost always medial; frequently associated with equinovarus deformity	Congenital: usually resolves itself; accelerate by close attention to sleeping position with extra diapers
	Muscular: strength imbalance in muscles attaching at knee joint, especially hamstrings (spina bifida)		Muscle imbalance: minimize through exercise and bracing such as derotation cables
	Movement pattern: linked pattern of hip and knee joint internal rotation, often in association with femoral anteversion (spastic cerebral palsy)		Movement pattern: anticipate emergence of mass internal rotation pattern; utilize muscle activation activites, weightbearing, and positioning to bias toward external rotation prior to achievement of walking
Hip			
Coxa Vara	Angle of inclination between femoral shaft and neck < 125°, possibly related to muscle pull imbalance	Femur oriented medially in the coronal plane in relation to the pelvis; leg shorter on affected side, with restricted abduction	Optimize alignment with shoe lift or ankle orthosis, depending on loading pattern and influence on knee

Table 3.1. continued

Name or Location	Pathology or Contributing Factors	Impairment; Associated Factors	Treatment
Coxa Valga	Failure of angle of inclination between femoral shaft and neck to decrease with growth from about 150°–125°	Femur oriented laterally in the coronal plane in relation to the pelvis; depending on foot orientation during loading, associated with genu varus and excessive hip abduction	May minimize impact on knee development and alignment through use of ankle orthosis; surgery required if hip dislocation also present
Dislocation	Congenital: external mechanical forces on joint, especially breech position during late gestation; sloping, shallow acetabulum; laxity of connective tissue in females; fetal akinesia syndrome	Hip may be subluxed in varying degrees to full dislocation; leg length difference indicative of dislocation; Barlow and Ortolani maneuvers identify subluxation	Congenital: multiple diapers, sleeping position, Pavlik harness, and Frejka pillow; conservative measures prior to walking; surgery sometimes necessary after 1 year
	Muscular: flaccid paralysis, minimal connective tissue support of the joint (spina bifida)		Muscular: positioning, weightbearing, and muscle activation; surgical repair of single dislocated hip to avoid scoliosis
	Movement pattern and tonal imbalance, shallow acetabulum, and deforming muscular pull on femur (spastic cerebral palsy)	Frequent association with chronic head and trunk asymmetry, exaggerated lower extremity stiffness, and hip adductor spasticity	Movement pattern: anticipate outcome in the presence of associated factors; utilize anticipatory positioning, tone decrement maneuvers, muscle activation, and early weightbearing

Table 3.1. continued

Name or Location	Pathology or Contributing Factors	Impairment; Associated Factors	Treatment
Femoral Anteversion	15° anteversion normal at maturity; conflicting accounts in literature as to whether anteversion or retroversion is prominent in infancy and early childhood	Excessive anterior orientation of femoral neck in relation to long axis of leg; increases hip internal rotation and tendency for in-toeing; often present with medial tibial rotation or torsion in spastic cerebral palsy	Anticipate development of excessive anteversion in spastic cerebral palsy; utilize alignment, tone decrement, and muscle activation maneuvers to attempt to balance muscle pull on developing hip and femur; surgical intervention occasionally necessary
Femoral Torsion	Spiraling within bone shaft of femur; may be normal in early infant development	Excessive spiraling may result from insufficient or excessive muscle pull influencing bone growth; often associated with femoral anteversion	Attempt to anticipate and balance muscle forces molding bone; surgical intervention often necessary in severe cases
Femoral Retroversion		Excessive posterior orientation of femoral neck in relation to long axis of leg; increases hip external rotation and tendency for out-toeing; may be diagnostic indicator of slipped capital femoral epiphysis in adolescent	

Table 3.1. continued

Name or Location	Pathology or Contributing Factors	Impairment; Associated Factors	Treatment
Trunk			
Pectus Carinatum	Fetal compression during gestation	Sternum elevated; chest has increased anterior-posterior dimensions	Improves with time and growth; no intervention in mild to moderately severe cases; surgery for cosmetic reasons in extreme instances
Pectus Excavatum	Gestational compression; shortened chorda tendineae of the diaphragm; chronic respiratory insufficiency, especially inspiratory stridor in premature infants	Sternum depressed relative to adjoining ribs	Identify and remediate cause of respiratory insufficiency; no specific intervention in mild to moderate cases; activation of abdominal musculature to elongate rib cage may have some value
Kyphosis	Occasionally due to skeletal disease, but frequently postural in relation to abnormally low or high muscle tone or paralysis	Trunk anterior curvature, usually accompanied by forward shoulders and forward or hyperextended head; thoracic or lumbar areas most common	Usually preventable by good attention to postural alignment by caregivers and selection of adaptive devices which promote best alignment
Scoliosis	Congenital: fetal positioning and confinement, especially in transverse position; Neuromusculoskeletal: unbalanced mechanical forces acting on	Trunk lateral curvature which may be accompanied by abnormal anterior-posterior alignment and vertebral and rib rotation; may be C-curve	Close attention to alignment, especially in supine and static sitting; exercises for general strengthening, elongation, and respiratory ca-

Table 3.1. continued

Name or Location	Pathology or Contributing Factors	Impairment; Associated Factors	Treatment
	developing spine due to paralysis or skeletal maldevelopment; Idiopathic: predisposing factors not obvious	or S-curve; may be functional (flexible) or structural (inflexible)	pacity; wide range of bracing, electrical stimulation, and surgical options; bracing or electrical stimulation indicated at 25°, surgery at 40°
Neck			
Torticollis	Fetal positioning or may develop postnatally due to excessive stretching during labor and delivery; may be early sign of generalized neuromotor abnormality	Exaggerated lateral flexion of head to one side and rotation to opposite side, often associated with shortening of one sternocleidomastoid muscle and plagiocephaly; may be associated with hypotonia or scoliosis	Musculoskeletal: good response to early intervention; promote supine sleeping with head rotated in opposite direction; gentle passive stretching and muscle activation efforts. Neuromuscular: identify source of asymmetry and remediate
Head			
Brachycephaly	Fetal constraint induced by early descent of fetal head into maternal pelvis; may be associated with genetic disorders such as Crouzon syndrome	Premature closure of coronal suture or both lambdoidal sutures; reduced anterior-posterior dimensions, head appears short, face retrusive; hypertelorism may be present	Early, corrective craniofacial surgery indicated in moderate to severe cases
Craniostenosis	Absence or limitation of growth stretch on a cranial suture line during gestation; may be secondary to defi-	Premature closure of one or several sutures; early, extensive closure due to fetal head entrapment in maternal	Early surgery indicated in moderate to severe cases for cosmetic reasons and to avoid impairment of brain growth

Table 3.1. continued

Name or Location	Pathology or Contributing Factors	Impairment; Associated Factors	Treatment
	cient brain growth	pelvis; may result in increased intracranial pressure	
Craniosynostosis	Premature suture closure often associated with genetic disorders rather than mechanical constraint	One or several sutures involved; frequently associated with other joint, facial deformities, hypertelorism	Craniofacial surgery indicated in moderate to severe cases for cosmetic reasons and to minimize brain impairment
Dolichocephaly	Fetal positioning; postnatal positioning exclusively in sidelying; premature closure of sagittal suture	Increased anterior-posterior, decreased lateral head dimensions, prominent forehead	May resolve without intervention, except for varied sleeping positions, depending on cause and severity
Plagiocephaly	Fetal constraint, often in association with torticollis (plagiocephaly-torticollis deformation sequence); asymmetrical premature suture closure; absence of varied sleeping positions for premature infants	Oblique molding of head with unilateral forehead prominence and contralateral occipital prominence; may be associated with ear, eye, neck, and trunk asymmetry	Spontaneous resolution may occur in 2–3 months, especially if neck alignment is treated; orthotic helmet is next measure, with neck exercises as noted above for torticollis; surgery may be indicated in severe cases
Scaphocephaly	Fetal confinement and high association with breech position	Flattened head, prominent occipital shelf, and increased anterior-posterior dimensions	Usually resolves without intervention, but varied sleeping positions required

Bronchopulmonary Dysplasia (BPD)

1. **Pathology:**
   a. Chronic pulmonary disease in infancy, typically preceded by infant respiratory distress syndrome (IRDS)
   b. Destruction of respiratory tract cilia and epithelium thought to be secondary to barotrauma from positive pressure ventilation and high oxygen administration
   c. May be accompanied by other conditions related to prematurity, such as intraventricular hemorrhage, necrotizing enterocolitis, and retinopathy of prematurity
2. **Impairment:**
   a. Respiratory support varies:
      - Complete mechanical ventilation may be required
      - Positive airway pressure methods may be used to maintain alveolar patency such as CPAP (continuous positive airway pressure) or PEEP (positive end expiratory pressure)
      - Nasal oxygen supplementation may be sufficient
   b. Majority of children are weaned from supplemental oxygen, but this process may take 2–3 years
   c. Motor developmental delay secondary to environmental limitations imposed by mechanical ventilation
3. **Functional Limitations:**
   a. Need for respiratory support equipment may require many months of hospitalization and, once home, radius of experience is limited by current ventilatory support
   b. In the absence of other disorders associated with prematurity, 3–6 months gross and fine motor developmental delay
4. **Treatment Goals and Interventions:**
   a. **Goal:** Promotion of gross and fine motor development
      - Specific gross and fine motor developmental interventions based on clinical findings and baseline standardized testing
      - Emphasis on midline and across midline skills requiring scapular protraction and trunk rotation; for example, child may be competent in static sitting, but not comfortable weightshifting across midline to bear weight on one arm and reach with the other
   b. **Goal:** Provide environmental adaptations to compensate for limitations imposed by respiratory support equipment
      - Fabricate or obtain devices to minimize specific limitations
      - For example, to promote midline fine motor function in sitting at home on the floor, fabricate a low table with a wide cutout to accommodate ventilator tubing in midline
   c. **Goal:** Increase endurance gradually
      - Treatment length and intensity should be designed to stay within child's cardiopulmonary limitations
      - Intensity of neuromotor interventions should be increased based on team interactions which address child's growth, nutritive needs, and cardiopulmonary maturation

Burns (Thermal Injuries)

1. **Pathology:**
   a. Partial or full-thickness soft tissue injuries due to contact with heat, chemical, or electrical agents
   b. If extensive, early hypovolemia and respiratory distress secondary to inhalation are life-threatening, as is infection later
   c. Skin injuries are most common, but burns of the respiratory tract and digestive tract also occur secondarily to inhalation and ingestion
   d. Extremity burns may be severe enough to lead to bone destruction and amputation
2. **Impairment:**
   a. Severe pain leading to immobility
   b. Early loss of skin elasticity due to pain, swelling, and skin grafting; later due to healing of skin and scarring in shortened joint position, also known as **position of comfort**
   c. Lack of mobility can lead to joint contractures, muscle atrophy, and diminished cardiopulmonary function
   d. Modified appearance following grafting or scarring may induce psychological stress
3. **Functional Limitations:** Loss of local and general mobility due to pain, swelling, loss of skin elasticity, joint contractures, and amputation in severe instances
4. **Treatment Goals and Interventions:**
   a. **Goal:** Attempt to maintain, rather than regain, range of motion
      - Very early joint mobility exercises carried out when child is heavily medicated can lay groundwork for effective maintenance of full range of motion throughout a long hospitalization
      - Promote teamwork among members of burn team so that early, sustained life-saving measures do not diminish awareness of need for daily range of motion exercises
      - Consult with child, family, and members of burn team to identify and provide opportunities for self-mobility even during acute stage
      - Develop early supportive relationship with child and family to counteract association with painful exercises
      - Utilize active and passive exercises to obtain full or optimal joint mobility whenever possible by coordinating with pain medication schedule
      - Do exactly what you say you will in terms of number of repetitions so that child can gain trust in you and sustain cooperation
      - Demonstrate high expectations for performance even in the presence of pain, but always finish session with something child wants
   b. **Goal:** Anticipate enormous physical and psychological stressors on child and family
      - Identify ways to give child and/or family control over scheduling of care procedures

- Identify child's preferences for food, recreation, or mobility and try to provide at least one per day
- Promote independence and a sense of competence in the child to demonstrate progression toward improvement

c. **Goal:** Optimal skin appearance and flexibility
- Cooperate with other caregivers to order custom elastic garments for skin compression to minimize scarring
- Fabricate skin contact thermoplastic splints, if needed, to promote optimal joint alignment and skin elongation during healing
- Promote very early **positions of function** before positions of comfort become firmly established, but avoid long periods of static positioning and immobility

5. Supplemental Interventions:

a. Skin debridement procedures and grafting early to minimize infection and hasten rehabilitation

b. Surgical release of skin and soft tissue contractures later to increase mobility of specific body segments

Calcaneovalgus (see Table 3.1)

Cardiac and Associated Vessel Anomalies in Infants and Children

1. Pathology:

a. Structural cardiovascular anomalies associated with arrested development occurring during gestational days 18–50

b. Rubella infection a documented cause, but maternal drug and alcohol ingestion, radiation exposure, other maternal infections, and maternal diabetes have also been suggested as contributory

c. Significant association with trisomy 21 or Down syndrome

2. Impairment:

a. **Patent ductus arteriosus:**
- Failure of ductus arteriosus to close soon after birth, allowing blood flow from high pressure aorta to pulmonary artery and a left to right shunt
- Often associated with prematurity
- Typically closed with medication, although surgery may be necessary
- Patency of this vessel may be maintained with medication (prostaglandins) to maintain life when more severe anomalies such as hypoplastic left heart syndrome or transposition of great vessels exist

b. **Atrial septal defect(s):**
- Single or multiple openings in the wall separating the two atria, decreasing blood flow going directly to ventricles and resulting in mild to moderate left to right shunt

- **Patent foramen ovale** most common atrial septal defect
- Often no intervention due to minimal impact on cardiodynamics and eventual closure over time

c. **Ventricular septal defect(s):**
- Single or multiple openings in the wall separating the ventricles, typically resulting in significant left to right shunt and transmission of the high pressures characteristic of the left heart to the pulmonary vascular bed
- Pulmonary engorgement results, minimizing the efficiency of oxygenation as a result of vessel engorgement
- Increasing pulmonary vascular resistance over time can create pulmonary hypertension and result in a right to left shunt, followed by cyanosis
- Surgical patching is almost always indicated

d. **Coarctation of the aorta:**
- Narrowing of the aorta in close approximation to the ductus arteriosus
- Increased resistance to blood flow in the left ventricle with decreased blood flow to the extremities
- Like **aortic stenosis,** may result in reopening of foramen ovale and creation of a left to right atrial shunt
- Surgical correction necessary for resolution

e. **Tetralogy of Fallot:**
- Includes **ventricular septal defect, pulmonary stenosis** and resulting **right ventricular hypertrophy, aortic dextroposition**
- Significant right to left shunt is the most common cause of cyanosis in children over 2 years of age
- Moderately severe exercise limitations until surgical correction is completed in stages

f. **Transposition of the great vessels:**
- Incomplete division of embryonic exit trunk from heart, resulting in aorta coming from right ventricle, and pulmonary artery from left
- Septal defects or patent ductus arteriosus necessary for continued vitality
- Cyanosis at rest and severe exercise restriction
- Surgical correction in stages may not lead to absence of limitations on exercise

g. **Hypoplastic left heart syndrome:**
- Left heart incapable of providing sufficient blood flow to maintain life
- Chemical maintenance of patency of ductus arteriosus or creation of atrial sepal defect sustains life until heart transplant can occur

3. Functional Limitations:

a. Exercise tolerance varies from no limitation to severe limitation with cyanosis at rest

b. Gross motor developmental delay very common in infants with severe anomalies, but relatively unresponsive to physical therapy interventions prior to corrective surgery

c. Pain and neck, thoracic, and shoulder movement limitation following surgery may result in life-threatening respiratory infection and joint mobility limitations

4. **Treatment Goals and Interventions:**
   a. **Goal:** Rule out other sources for developmental delay and select interventions appropriate for child's developmental level and cardiorespiratory status
      - Confirm signs of cardiorespiratory distress for a specific child with physician and family
      - Utilize age-appropriate activities for intervention well within child's level of tolerance
      - Communicate with all caregivers regarding limited expectations for motor developmental change prior to surgical intervention
      - Select and utilize assistive devices to foster independent function

   b. **Goal:** Obtain full neck, shoulder, and thoracic range of motion and pulmonary clearance following surgery in association with other caregivers
      - Evaluate child's postural alignment and neck, shoulder, and chest range of motion preoperatively and postoperatively, and intervene with gentle exercises and postural correction as needed
      - Assess coughing, demonstrate coughing, postural drainage, vibration, compression, and percussion preoperatively and follow through postoperatively if indicated with collaboration of other caretakers; discuss intranasal suctioning preoperatively
      - Cooperate with child, family, and other caretakers to identify best means of achieving optimal pulmonary hygiene and gas exchange following surgery

   c. **Goal:** Evaluate gross and fine motor development postoperatively when child has recovered from surgical intervention and develop intervention program linked with assessment findings
      - In collaboration with physician and family, utilize fairly aggressive intervention measures to accelerate gross and fine motor performance within child's level of physical and psychological tolerance
      - Identify child's and family's priorities for intervention activities to be incorporated into intervention program

5. **Supplemental Interventions:**
   a. Closure of septal defects and patent ductus arteriosus (**PDA**) with drugs and surgical patching
   b. Creation or maintenance of patency with drugs or surgical intervention may be necessary to sustain life
   c. Closed heart surgery for stenotic valves, coarctation of the aorta, ligation of PDA; open heart surgery for all other listed anomalies
   d. **Heart transplantation** followed by chemical immunosuppression for hypoplastic left heart syndrome and transposition of great vessels in some cases
   e. **Heart and lung transplantation** followed by immunosuppression indicated for pulmonary vascular disease or inadequate pulmonary arteries

Cardiac Defects (see Cardiac Anomalies)

Cavus Foot (Pes Cavus) (see Table 3.1)

Cerebral Palsy

1. Pathology:

a. Group of disorders prenatal, perinatal, or postnatal in origin
b. Static encephalopathy which may lead to development of progressive neuromusculoskeletal limitations
c. May result from infection, trauma, cranial hypoxia, or consanguinity
d. Frequently associated with placental insufficiency, prematurity, Grade III or IV intraventricular hemorrhage

2. Impairment:

a. **Spastic Cerebral Palsy:**
- Increased muscle tone, typically in antigravity musculature
- Muscle imbalance across joints may lead to range of motion limitations of scapular protraction and depression, glenohumeral flexion, abduction, external rotation, elbow, wrist and finger extension, forearm supination, hip abduction, extension, external rotation, knee extension, ankle dorsiflexion, and supination

b. **Spastic Quadriplegia:**
- Four extremity involvement, as well as throat, neck, and trunk musculature
- Neonatal feeding dyscoordination and generalized hypotonia may be first symptoms; if present, low tone gradually transitions to muscle imbalance and spasticity over the 1st year
- Early neuromotor indicators for treatment: very erect head position in prone accompanied by poor ability to flex or right head in supine, elbows flexed and positioned well behind shoulders in prone accompanied by inability to reach or extend hands to midline in supine, little isolated finger motion, extended legs with minimal ankle dorsiflexion
- Same symptoms are also present with **transient dystonia,** which resolves at about 1 year of age
- May be associated with seizures, hip subluxation, cognitive, visual, auditory, and oral motor deficits

c. **Spastic Diplegia:**
- Mainly lower extremity involvement
- Gait characterized by short stride length, excessive hip adduction and internal rotation, and ankle plantar flexion
- Lower extremity reciprocal movements in crawling and dissociation in all positions difficult to attain
- High association with prematurity
- May be associated with oral motor and visual deficits

d. **Spastic Hemiplegia:**
   - One side of the body affected, especially trunk and extremities
   - Child's tendency is often to disregard affected side and compensate with opposite side
   - Rarely motor milestone delay
   - Equinus deformity secondary to tendo-achilles shortening a common complication, which can be minimized by early, auticipatory treatment
   - Increased effort with unaffected side may elicit associated reactions: upper extremity scapular retraction, shoulder external rotation, elbow flexion, lower extremity adduction, internal rotation, and plantar flexion
   - May be associated with strabismus, seizures, speech, learning, and perceptual disorders

e. **Ataxic Cerebral Palsy:**
   - Generalized decreased muscle tone; infant may initially be diagnosed with "floppy baby syndrome"
   - Wide base of support (BOS) characteristic in weight bearing positions
   - Ataxia and dyscoordination elicited by decreased BOS as the child assumes more erect positions
   - Hip abduction contractures occasionally present
   - May be associated with poor visual tracking and speech delay
   - High association with abnormal cerebellar development

f. **Athetoid Cerebral Palsy:**
   - Most common type of dyskinetic cerebral palsy
   - Extraneous movements associated with postural instability and fluctuating muscle tone, particularly apparent during speech, feeding, and upper extremity activities
   - High association with erythroblastosis secondary to maternal-infant Rh incompatibility and hyperbilirubinemia
   - Cognitive ability typically within normal range
   - Hearing loss may be present

g. **Mixed Cerebral Palsy:** usually denotes presence of athetosis and spasticity, but may be used to describe other combinations

h. **Other:** rare types of cerebral palsy which do not correspond to above categories, including other types of dyskinetic CP or atonic CP, which may be transitional in young infant and later become spastic or athetoid cerebral palsy

3. Functional Limitations:

a. Dependent on type of cerebral palsy

b. Range of motion limitations may restrain mobility of children with spasticity

c. Walking without aids achieved by children with hemiplegia and some children with diplegia or ataxia; walking with canes, crutches, or rollator walker achieved by children with diplegia, some with athetosis, and a few children with quadriplegia

d. Hypotonia and joint hypermobility with ataxia may decrease with age and increasing level of function

e. Independence in oral motor and manipulatory skills typically achieved by children with hemiplegia and mild to moderate diplegia

4. **Goals and Interventions:** highly individualized treatment depending on child's abilities, age, type of cerebral palsy, and associated conditions
   a. **Goal:** Maximize development of movement capabilities and avoid contractures
      - Intervene early with mobility and developmental activities in response to subtle signs of muscle imbalance in infants: axial extensor muscle dominance accompanied by poor neck and anterior trunk flexor function, chronic asymmetrical posture, fisted hands in associated with scapular retraction, and stiff legs with little ankle motion
      - Simulate age-appropriate gross and fine motor experiences if the child is unable to do this
         - Initiate standing through supported weightbearing by 9–10 months
         - Provide trunk and upper extremity alignment through appropriate positioning to facilitate the development of manipulatory and feeding skills
         - Facilitate child's efforts to initiate or complete transitions between positions, such as sidelying to sitting or sitting to quadruped

   b. **Goal:** Address oral motor function in the context of child's total motor function
      - In conjunction with speech and occupational therapy, identify and utilize nipples, spoons, and other feeding devices to improve oral motor function
      - Utilize seating or other positional devices to provide optimal alignment for eating and communication

   c. **Goal:** Identify and respond to tone abnormality in order to increase opportunities for self-initiated movements
      - Utilize static (positional) and dynamic rotation to decrease high truncal and extremity tone in order to promote the emergence of motor behaviors which may not occur in the presence of high tone
      - To increase very low tone, avoid static rotational positions and utilize extremity loading (weightbearing) and postural challenges to increase positional stability

   d. **Goal:** Minimize or prevent sequelae to early alignment or neuromotor problems through early intervention
      - Minimize or correct early head and truncal asymmetry which may precede scoliosis and hip dislocation
      - Emphasize elongation of hip adductors and internal rotators to promote wide base of support and increased stride length in a child with spasticity
      - Emphasize elongation of spastic hamstrings to minimize tendency toward kyphosis and posterior pelvic tilt in child with spasticity
      - Utilize generalized trunk and neck strengthening exercises to improve stability and back alignment in child with low tone and ataxia
      - Utilize sidelying positioning in adduction and extremity loading through kneeling or standing to minimize tendency for iliotibial band tightness in children with hypotonia

e. **Goal:** Integrate interventions into child's daily caretaking activities in order to maximize educational and neuromotor outcomes
   - Work together with the child, parents, and caretakers in child's environment to achieve consensus on positioning, equipment, and dynamic interventions linked to specific goals
   - Determine child's and parents' goals as primary goals
   - Identify environmental limitations which may require compensation so that child functions optimally; for example, access to neighborhood school may be an obstacle to getting to child's classroom, or parents' other responsibilities may limit amount of time child can stand in a supine stander at home on weekdays

5. Supplemental Interventions for Cerebral Palsy:

a. **Direct Muscle Stimulation:** Preliminary evidence based on case reports of 5 children suggests that neuromuscular electrical stimulation (NMES) in conjunction with a task-oriented physical therapy program may result in functional gains related to the muscle group stimulated

b. **Neurosurgical:**
   - **Spinal Cord Stimulation (SCS):** Electrical stimulation of the spinal cord via electrodes placed on the dura mater has been shown to alter, principally to reduce, spasticity
   - **Selective Dorsal Rhizotomy:**
     - Surgical procedure to reduce spasticity; following lumbar laminectomy
     - Electrical stimulation to dorsal rootlets produces EMG responses
     - Those rootlets associated with abnormal EMG responses are severed
     - Daily or 3 times weekly physical therapy for several weeks following surgery is desirable for optimal outcome, as weakness following surgery is common
     - Long-term results are unavailable and the risks and benefits of this surgery have not been clearly determined

c. **Pharmaceutical:**
   - Oral or intrathecal baclofen introduced into the spinal cord may decrease spasticity or involuntary movements in children and adults
   - Intrathecal baclofen has fewer side effects; these include hypotonia, attention deficit, sedation, and enuresis.
   - Dantrolene sodium has also been reported to decrease spasticity, but functional changes have not been documented
   - Phenol injections into specific muscles, especially the gastroc-soleus complex, have been associated with short-term reduction in spasticity

d. **Orthopedic:**
   - **Casting and Bracing** decisions are generally made by the physical therapist in conjunction with an orthopedist or physiatrist
   - **Casting options** include: (1) serial casting to regain lost range of motion (2) casting designed to change muscle tone and length relationships in the leg or arm through passive positioning of 1 or more joints; may be solid or bivalve (3) cast-

ing designed to improve alignment and stability distally in order to concentrate on improving proximal muscle control; typically bivalve, used during treatment sessions; ski boots are commonly used for this purpose in Switzerland (4) casting following bony surgery or soft tissue releases; rarely, casting following scoliosis surgery (5) casting to assess response to realignment which may assist in a bracing decision

- **Bracing:** Custom-molded thermoplastic orthoses are typical; range of options:
  - Submalleolar orthoses address forefoot and midfoot alignment
  - Supramalleolar orthoses limit calcaneal eversion or inversion
  - Articulated MAFO's (molded ankle-foot orthoses) maintain optimal foot alignment and encourage dorsiflexion beyond neutral while limiting plantar flexion
  - Rigid MAFO's maintain the ankle close to a 90° angle
  - Braces higher than AFO's very rare because of the coordination and strength required to move them; however, a pelvic band is occasionally used with twister cables mounted laterally on AFO's as a derotational alignment assist during gait
  - Dynamic ankle-foot orthoses (DAFO's) typically extend to low or midcalf and are fabricated with less rigid materials
- **Surgery:** ranges from percutaneous tendon lengthening to bone reconstruction

Congenital Hip Dislocation (see Table 3.1)

Coxa Vara, Coxa Valga (see Table 3.1)

Craniostenosis (see Table 3.1)

Craniosynostosis (see Table 3.1)

Cystic Fibrosis

1. **Pathology:**
   a. Inherited progressive disorder of the exocrine glands transmitted according to an autosomal recessive pattern in which both parents are carriers
   b. 25% chance that offspring will be affected
   c. Pancreatic insufficiency, hyperplasia of mucous-producing cells in the lungs, excessive electrolyte secretion by the sweat glands, which is the basis for diagnosis using the sweat test, and digital clubbing
2. **Impairment:**
   a. Incomplete digestion and nutritional insufficiency, which can be addressed with pancreatic enzyme supplementation

b. Production of thick, excessive pulmonary secretions which are the source of airway obstruction and chronic lung infection
c. Limited rib excursion, use of accessory muscles of respiration, barrel chest deformity
d. Pneumothorax and hemoptysis may be late manifestations

3. **Functional Limitations:**
   a. Dependent on age and extent of gastrointestinal (GI) and pulmonary involvement; for example, GI problems may be remediated by enzyme supplements only or may require nighttime intraesophageal tube feeding
   b. Endurance limited by pulmonary involvement can range from some participation in a team sport such as swimming to maximal oxygen supplementation needed for ambulation
4. **Goals and Interventions:**
   a. **Goal:** Bronchial hygiene: removal of airway secretions
      - Aerosol medications to promote drainage
      - Postural drainage positions for all lung areas with emphasis on those identified as congested with auscultation
      - Percussion, vibration with expiration, and deep coughing with expectoration

   b. **Goal:** Chest wall mobility
      - Minimize hyperinflation by consistent bronchial hygiene
      - Breathing exercises to maintain balanced proportions of rib cage
      - Positioning, relaxation, and retraining to minimize use of accessory muscles of respiration

   c. **Goal:** Optimal postural alignment: through exercises and postural awareness, anticipate and avoid or minimize forward head, elevated and forward shoulders, and kyphosis and scoliosis
   d. **Goal:** Cardiopulmonary conditioning
      - Except in severe disease, identify, with the child, appropriate sports and recreational activities
      - Swimming has been shown to facilitate clearing of secretions
5. **Supplemental Interventions:**
   a. Hyperalimentation during the night frequently used to improve nutritional status
   b. Medications to enhance digestion and combat infections significant aspects of treatment
   c. Recently developed, genetically engineered drug, DNAse (Dornase alfa), a.k.a. Pulmozyme, appears to decrease incidence of chronic respiratory infection in cystic fibrosis

Dolichocephaly (see Table 3.1)

Down syndrome (Trisomy 21)

1. **Pathology:**
   a. Genetic disorder usually associated with an extra 21st chromosome due to nondisjunction occurring prior to fertilization
   b. Can also result from translocation of chromosomal material following breakage
   c. Mild form associated with mosaicism, in which some cells have trisomy 21 and others have a normal chromosomal complement
   d. Phenotype, or physical appearance, of children with mosaicism more closely resembles child without the facial features associated with Down syndrome
   e. Has been described as the most common pattern of human malformation and one of most common causes of cognitive delay
2. **Impairment:** Diagnosis is generally made shortly after birth based on the presence of 4–6 of the following features: hypotonia, poor Moro response, joint hyperflexibility, excess skin on the back of the neck, flat facial profile, upslanted palpebral fissures, external ear anomalies, pelvic hypoplasia with shallow acetabular angle, dysplasia of midphalanx of 5th finger, and Simian crease (single midpalmar crease)
   a. **Neurological:**
      - Generalized hypotonia most consistent finding
      - Motor delay as well as delayed speech acquisition associated with hypotonia
      - Correlation between hypotonia and cognitive delay also reported
   b. **Cardiopulmonary:**
      - Cardiac anomalies are present in 40% of individuals with Down syndrome and may independently contribute to gross motor delay
      - Ventricular septal defects and atrioventricular canal defects most common and usually repaired surgically during infancy
   c. **Auditory and Visual:**
      - Hearing and visual deficits are both common in children with Down syndrome
      - Incidence of each ranges from 40–60%
      - Otitis media is prevalent and a frequent source of hearing loss
   d. **Musculoskeletal:**
      - Atlanto-axial subluxation or dislocation as a result of ligamentous laxity identified in 12–20% of individuals with Down syndrome
      - Orthopedic evaluation by 2 years of age and avoidance of sports which include vigorous neck flexion and rotation activities recommended
      - Other orthopedic problems associated with hypotonicity and hyperflexibility, in decreasing order of occurrence, include: pes planus, metatarsus varus, scoliosis, patellar subluxation or dislocation, and hip subluxation or dislocation
   e. **Cognitive:**
      - Smaller brain size, reduced head circumference, and a less complex gyral pattern may be related to significant cognitive deficit associated with disorder
      - Additional microscopic findings include: abnormal synaptic morphology, particularly synaptic spines, and decreased synaptogenesis

- Probable migration defect of smaller neurons and myelination delay
- Pyramidal neuron abnormalities identified in several sites thought to be associated with cognitive and motor delay

3. Functional Limitations:

a. Hypotonia and delayed acquisition of antigravity postural responses contribute to gross motor delay

b. Cognitive and perceptual deficits may contribute to delays in fine motor, cognitive, and psychosocial development

c. Tongue protrusion, hypotonia, and difficulty maintaining mouth closure are bases for feeding difficulties and delayed onset of speech

d. Cardiopulmonary function is an exercise limitation prior to surgery and, rarely, after surgery in children with cardiac anomalies

e. Forceful neck flexion and rotation activities should be avoided in order to minimize risk of C1–C2 dislocation

f. If permitted to develop, obesity has negative impact on the schedule of attainment of gross motor skills

4. Treatment Goals and Interventions:

a. **Goal:** In conjunction with speech and occupational therapy, promote effective oral motor function by encouraging tongue retrusion and lip closure

- Through appropriate nipple choice and/or infant's and parent's body position during early infancy, achieve adequate nipple seal and efficient sucking
- Utilize gentle tactile cues; for example, horizontally oriented forefinger pressure just below the lower lip and imitation such as kissing or puckering encourages mouth closure at appropriate times
- Introduce sucking with a straw before transition from bottle to cup is complete
- Promote straw use for obtaining most liquids

b. **Goal:** Anticipate gross and fine motor delay and provide antigravity interventions to minimize it

- Utilize positioning and weightshifting activities in prone during early infancy to facilitate head elevation and rotation, upper extremity weightbearing, reaching, prone circular pivoting, and rolling from prone to supine
- Provide overhead activities and toys in supine and supported semi-sitting to promote reaching, eye-hand coordination, and midline manual activity
- Develop neck and anterior trunk antigravity competence through elicited rolling from supine to sidelying and gentle, small arc pull-to-sit activities with head support
- Emphasize trunk extension and extremity loading activities which tend to increase axial tone; avoid emphasis on body flexion activities which generally reduce tone
- Introduce sitting opportunities when chronologically appropriate if head control is sufficient
- Introduce dynamic rather than static positional, standing experience when chronologically appropriate if trunk stability and ankle alignment permit

c. **Goal:** Anticipate delayed antigravity postural responses: provide opportunities for postural response practice integrated with functional activities which have a cognitive or fine motor component
d. **Goal:** Using appropriate equipment, provide optimal body alignment to support gross, fine, and oral motor progress and cognitive development
   - In consultation with parents and speech and occupational therapists, identify sitting devices and positions which promote success with fine motor and cognitive tasks and optimize oral motor function
   - UCBL submalleolar or supramalleolar orthoses may be needed to **ensure** appropriate foot alignment during early standing

Equinovarus Foot (see Table 3.1)

Equinus Foot (see Table 3.1)

Femoral Anteversion, Retroversion, or Torsion (see Table 3.1)

Genu Recurvatum (see Table 3.1)

Genu Valgus (see Table 3.1)

Genu Varus, Tibia Vara or Blount Disease (see Table 3.1)

Hip Dislocation (see Table 3.1)

Hemophilia:

1. **Pathology:** X-linked recessive disorder resulting in impaired blood clotting capability; females are carriers
   a. **Hemophilia A:** Factor VIII deficiency which can be identified through fetal blood typing at 18–20 weeks' gestational age
   b. **Hemophilia B:** Factor IX deficiency which can be identified by DNA analysis following amniocentesis or chorionic villus biopsy
   c. Differentiate from **von Willebrand's Disease,** autosomal disorder characterized by superficial bleeding into mucocutaneous tissues and occurrence in females
   d. Significantly high occurrence of **HIV** and **AIDS** in individuals with hemophilia due to unintended transfusion of infected blood products prior to identification of virus in the blood supply
2. **Impairment:**
   a. Pain and reduced range of motion and muscle strength in joints into which bleeding occurs **(hemarthrosis)**
   b. Hinge joints most typically affected: knee, elbow, and ankle
   c. Intracranial hemorrhage can occur, leading to death

d. Encapsulated hematomas, **pseudotumors,** requiring surgical removal can occur adjacent to bones following intramuscular hemorrhages

3. **Functional Limitations:**
   a. Loss of joint specific or general mobility following bleeding
   b. Chronic arthritis can occur in response to many hemorrhages into the same joint
4. **Treatment Goals and Interventions**
   a. **Goal:** Cooperate with treatment team to minimize joint and other hemorrhages
   - Promote patient and family education with respect to blood replacement products
     - **Replacement therapy** with Factor VIII is most common, but Factors II, VII, IX, X, and XIII also utilized in a cryoprecipitate medium
     - Patients occasionally develop **factor inhibitors** which are suspected if bleeding episode does not respond to replacement therapy
   - Evidence suggests that early, proactive muscle strengthening exercises in young boys may exert protective effect on their muscles and joints
   - Identify, with child and family, sports and other recreational activities to promote optimal cardiopulmonary fitness, strengthening, and mobility
   - May wish to avoid contact sports such as football or hockey

   b. **Goal:** Participate in appropriate response to joint or muscle hemorrhage
   - Hematoma treated with elastic pressure bandage and ice
   - Joint may be immobilized for 1–2 days following bleeding, utilizing previously or currently fabricated temporary splint
   - Reintroduce mobility through exercise appropriate for symptoms and level of function

Joint Deformations (see Table 3.1)

Joint Deformations Related to Fetal Position or Confinement

1. **Pathology:**
   a. Isolated joint deformations result from fetal positioning in utero or uterine confinement
   b. Female infants more susceptible, possibly due to estrogenic ligamentous laxity; male infants may be spared due to toughening effect of testosterone on connective tissue
   c. Contributing factors: primigravida (first pregnancy), small maternal size, uterine malformation or tumor, insufficient amniotic fluid (oligohydramnios), fetal crowding associated with multiple births, and atypical fetal position
   d. **Multiple** congenital joint contractures more often associated with neuromuscular pathology and fetal akinesia syndrome (discussed under **Multiple Congenital Contractures** or **Arthrogryposis**)
2. **Impairment:** Foot deformities most common, although congenital hip dislocation, tibial torsion, genu recurvatum, pectus excavatum, pectus carinatum, and scoliosis may also occur (see Table 3.1 for specific descriptions)

3. **Functional Limitations (Foot Deformities):** limitations range from no impact on gait with or without orthotic compensation to decreased gait velocity and postural stability to jump off of and land on foot
4. **Treatment Goals and Interventions:**
   a. **Goal:** Optimal or improved joint alignment
   b. Interventions (see Table 3.1)

Juvenile Rheumatoid Arthritis (JRA)

1. **Pathology:**
   a. Group of diseases characterized by chronic joint inflammation
   b. Specific pathology unknown, but thought to be an autoimmune disorder in response to infection or trauma in an individual with genetic predisposition
   c. May resolve spontaneously
   d. Several subtypes
2. **Impairment:**
   a. **Systemic JRA:**
      - Multisystem involvement in addition to multiple joint pain and inflammation
      - May include pericarditis, myocarditis, hepatosplenomegaly, and other organ involvement
      - Equal distribution in males and females
   b. **Polyarticular JRA:**
      - Involvement of 5 or more joints, usually symmetrical distribution
      - Knees and ankles frequently involved; elbows, wrists, and fingers less often; temporomandibular joint and cervical spine rarely
      - More prominent in girls
   c. **Pauciarticular JRA:** most frequently occurring type with joint involvement in 4 joints or fewer; 2 subgroups:
      - Females age 4 years or less:
        - High risk of blindness secondary to chronic inflammation of iris **(iridocyclitis)**
        - Biannual ophthalmologic monitoring necessary even if joint disease resolves
      - Males predominantly age 10 years or more; typically have hip joint involvement which may progress to pelvis and spine
3. **Functional Limitations:**
   a. Dependent on pain and specific or generalized joint mobility limitations and involvement of other organ systems
   b. Gait usually affected through diminished velocity and stride length with antalgic character
   c. Crutches or modified walker use may be necessary to maintain ambulation
   d. Elbow, wrist, and finger inflammation and reduced mobility may severely affect ability to carry out daily activities independently

4. **Treatment Goals and Interventions:**
   a. **Goal:** Attain and maintain optimal joint mobility and muscle strength
      - Encourage continued participation in exercise program through selection of activities that incorporate child's and family's interests
      - Utilize concurrent multiple joint exercise strategies rather than isolated joint exercises whenever feasible
      - Identify recreational or social means of achieving optimal joint mobility and strength to minimize emphasis on disability
      - Select activities for physical therapy sessions that are difficult or impossible to do in other settings to minimize redundancy
      - Incorporate muscle strengthening activities which minimize joint destruction or pain; isometrics may be preferred by patient and therapist
   b. **Goal:** Monitor joint alignment carefully and intervene as necessary to promote optimal alignment
      - Anticipate deformations such as genu valgus and ulnar drift, which are often associated with rheumatoid arthritis
         - Avoid range of motion exercises which contribute to these tendencies
         - Selectively bias joints by exercising in opposing directions before deformations occur
      - Selection of specific trunk or extremity elongation or postural activities to optimize alignment, especially if embedded in recreational pursuit, is often far more effective than verbal cues to improve posture
   c. **Goal:** Participate actively in teamwork decisions to obtain optimal outcome for child in the context of family
      - Identify child and family's treatment and other priorities
      - Communicate with caregivers in multiple settings to ensure consistency in family interactions and care
      - Encourage consideration of needs of siblings and ensure that they are not overlooked by family members or caregivers
5. **Supplementary Interventions:** Medical management is a priority. Effective medication choices can significantly minimize joint inflammation and mobility limitations as well as reduce other systemic manifestations.

Kyphosis (see Table 3.1)

Leg Length Discrepancy: an outcome not related to a specific pathological process:

- **Congenital:** secondary to hip dislocation, hemimelia in which 1 segment is shorter, or hemihypertrophy in which 1 side of the body is larger
- **Acquired:** secondary to paralysis, vascular differences in each leg, neoplasm, especially Wilm's tumor, growth plate damage as a result of trauma or fracture

1. **Impairment:**
   a. **True** leg length discrepancy is within the leg
      - Often evident on visual comparison of femoral lengths in supine with hips and knees in 90° of flexion (one knee higher) or Galeazzi sign: tibial-fibial lengths with hips and knees flexed and feet flat on the surface (1 knee higher)
      - Measurement from ASIS to medial malleolus is different and in standing, a block under 1 foot is necessary to level the pelvis

   b. **Apparent** leg length discrepancy frequently due to pelvic obliquity associated with scoliosis, or hip abduction or flexion contracture, but may also be result of knee or ankle contracture. Measurement from the xiphoid process to medial malleolus different on each side
2. **Functional Limitations:**
   a. None if difference is less than 1/2 in
   b. If greater, gait and postural alignment may be negatively affected and potential for development of deformities with continuing growth exists
3. **Treatment Goals and Interventions:**
   a. **Goal:** Discriminate unequivocally between real and apparent leg length discrepancy: use assessment methods described above and others as needed
   b. **Goal:** Achieve postural symmetry through compensatory strategies. In conjunction with an orthopedist, determine whether shoe lift, orthotic modification, exercises to improve limited joint mobility or postural alignment, or interventions beyond the scope of physical therapy are indicated to achieve symmetry

Metatarsus Adductus (see Table 3.1)

Multiple Congenital Contractures (formerly called Arthrogryposis Multiplex Congenita)

1. **Pathology:**
   a. Joint contractures due to intrauterine akinesia or dyskinesia may be outcome of more than 100 conditions typically associated with neurological, muscle, or connective tissue disease
   b. Fetal crowding and fetal constraint with multiple births also contributory
   c. Significant association with breech position and oligohydramnios (reduced volume of amniotic fluid)
2. **Impairment:**
   a. Multiple, nonprogressive, symmetrical joint contractures in infants, often accompanied by hip dislocation, club feet, and generalized muscle atrophy
   b. Deep tendon reflexes absent or reduced
   c. Sensation intact
   d. No intellectual impairment
   e. Joint mobility improves with age

3. **Functional Limitations:**
   a. Ambulation and manipulation frequently require assistive devices
   b. Endurance may be limited related to effort of walking
4. **Treatment Goals and Interventions:**
   a. **Goal:** Increase range of motion: exercises, serial casting, or splinting begin in neonatal period
   b. **Goal:** Optimal lower extremity alignment by 2 years of age: above interventions may be supplemented with motor developmental activities, surgery for club feet, joint contracture or hip dislocation, and preambulatory weightbearing with standing devices
   c. **Goal:** Maximal independence in activities of daily living
      - Exercises, splinting, and surgery to increase upper extremity range of motion and strength
      - Adaptive devices to facilitate eating, daily care activities, and walking
   d. **Goal:** Maximal opportunity for cognitive and social development: consider early choices of mobility-enhancement devices to promote independent exploration and socialization

Muscular Dystrophy (see Table 3.2)

Myopathies (see Table 3.2)

Myotonic Dystrophy (see Table 3.2)

Myelomeningocele (see Spina Bifida)

Osteogenesis Imperfecta (see Chapter 1)

Pectus Carinatum (see Table 3.1)

Pectus Excavatum (see Table 3.1)

Plagiocephaly (see Table 3.1)

Rheumatoid Arthritis (see Juvenile Rheumatoid Arthritis)

Scaphocephaly (see Table 3.1)

Scoliosis (see Table 3.1)

Sickle Cell Disease (Anemia)

1. **Pathology:**
   a. Autosomal recessive disorder most prominent in individuals of African descent
   b. Genetic trait which protects against malaria in Africa promotes sickle cell disease in U.S. and Europe

Table 3.2. Intrinsic Muscle Diseases

Myopathy	Pathology	Impairment	Functional Limitations	Treatment Goals (G) and Interventions (I) For All Disorders
Duchenne's Muscular Dystrophy (DMD or Pseudohypertrophic Muscular Dystrophy)	Inherited by males as an X-linked recessive; females rarely affected, but are carriers; pseudohypertropic calf muscles common; intrinsic muscle disease, not an anterior horn cell disorder; CK elevated, dystrophin absent	Progressive, intrinsic muscle weakness by 3 years of age; progressing to death in late adolescence or early adulthood; weakness from proximal to distal; Gower's maneuver compensates for quadriceps and gluteal weakness	Delayed motor milestones; loss of ambulation leading to wheelchair use; may be nonprogressive cognitive deficit; joint mobility limitations; progressive cardiopulmonary limitation	**G: Parent education** I: Inform parents of existence and role of genetic counseling if child has a genetic disorder & they are in childbearing years **G: Maintain mobility as long as possible** I: Encourage functional activities rather than specific strengthening regimens I: Utilize adaptive equipment to promote maximum independence I: Encourage recreational activities to optimize quality of life experiences I: Promote cardiopul-
Becker Muscular Dystrophy	Allelic, milder variant of DMD; level of dystrophin reduced rather than absent	Onset of weakness 5–15 years or later, proximal to distal progression	Motor milestones may be normal; ambulation maintained to 25–45 years of age	
Limb-Girdle Muscular Dystrophy (Erb's Dystrophy)	Autosomal recessive; diverse group of disorders in males and females characterized by proximal weakness	Onset of weakness in 2nd decade; slow progression from proximal to distal; pattern of weakness more generalized than DMD	Determined by age of onset and rate of progression; stability of gait may be decreased only slightly to full loss of ambulation	

Table 3.2. continued

Myopathy	Pathology	Impairment	Functional Limitations	Treatment Goals (G) and Interventions (I) For All Disorders
Facioscapulohumeral (Landouzy-Dejerine) Muscular Dystrophy	Autosomal dominant disorder in females and males; severe form may present in infants as Moebius syndrome or sequence	Onset of weakness at any age, especially after 2nd decade; initial involvement in face and shoulder girdle, progresses to pelvic girdle; asymmetrical weakness	Mild course; many families do not consider it problematic; severe form may be associated with hearing loss, speech impairment, feeding problems, and early onset of disability	monary fitness through activities of daily living and recreation **G: Anticipate contractures** I: Utilize positioning devices to attain optimal alignment and to minimize need for painful stretching I: Select positioning devices which promote maximal mobility, rather than static positioning which leads to reduced fitness
Myotonic Dystrophy (Steinert Syndrome)	Autosomal dominant disorder with variable penetrance; males and females; characterized by distal weakness; gene defect identified on chromosome 19; cataracts and cardiac conduction anomalies	Absence or weakness of sternocleidomastoid muscle; weakness progresses distally to proximally; myotonia refers to sustained contraction following effort; variable onset from birth–5th decade	Congenital form associated with facial weakness, feeding, and speech difficulties; motor milestones delayed, but good potential for ambulation; cognitive impairment; cardiopulmonary limitations	

Table 3.2. continued

Myopathy	Pathology	Impairment	Functional Limitations	Treatment Goals (G) and Interventions (I) For All Disorders
Central Core Myopathy	Autosomal dominant congenital myopathy; decreased mitochrondria and enzyme activity; central cores in type I fibers	Weakness usually nonprogressive; generalized hypotonia (floppy baby)	Motor milestone delay; mild to moderate weakness later; general picture is improvement; early respiratory support common	
Nemaline Myopathy	Autosomal dominant, variable penetrance, males and females; cardiac involvement may occur; nemaline rods in continuity with z-band	Variable onset, infancy to childhood; weakness nonprogressive or slowly progressive; marked hypotonia and/or arachnodactyly may be present	Motor milestone delay; mild to moderate weakness later; benign course unless cardiac involvement which may be fatal	
Myotubular Myopathy	Autosomal recessive or X-linked recessive, male and female distribution depends on genetic cause	Onset in infancy; hypotonia; ptosis, facial, and optical paralysis; slow progression of weakness	Moderate to severe weakness present in adolescence permits limited ambulation; joint contractures limit mobility	

c. Red blood cells (RBC's) assume crescent shape because altered hemoglobin (hemoglobin S) forms long crystalline aggregates when deoxygenated; aggregates distort the RBC's into a crescent or sickle shape promoting excessive clustering
d. Neurological complications secondary to cell clusters

2. **Impairment:**
   a. **Pain related to sickle cell crisis:** intense localized muscle and joint pain and possibly painful penile erections (priapism)
   b. **Hemiplegia:** paralysis or paresis secondary to embolic-like cell clusters
3. **Functional Limitations:**
   a. Limited respiratory reserve; avoid cardiorespiratory challenges
   b. Severity of hemiplegia may affect bilateral hand function, and gait stability and velocity
4. **Treatment Goals and Interventions:**
   a. **Goal:** Identify and minimize behaviors which may lead to sickle cell crises
      - Avoid high demand cardiorespiratory challenges
      - Identify and select devices to support functional independence in face of restrictions
   b. **Goal:** Treat discomfort related to sickle cell crisis; intervene only after discussion with physician and in response to specific symptoms with established physical therapy procedures for muscle and joint pain
   c. **Goal:** Respond to neurological complications such as hemiplegia
      - Following assessment, provide tone decrement and muscle activation strategies to obtain optimal alignment, joint mobility, and dynamic motor function
      - Select assistive devices as needed to improve gait and upper extremity function

Spina Bifida

1. **Pathology:**
   a. Spinal cord and/or vertebral malformation, usually thoracic or lumbar, as a result of neural tube defect
   b. Failure of closure of superior neural tube (neuropore) at 3–4 weeks' gestational age results in **anencephaly**
   c. Failure of closure of inferior neuropore at 3–4 weeks' gestational age results in **spina bifida**
   d. Increasing evidence for link between maternal hot soaking baths and neural tube defects and protective role of folic acid and/or beta carotene supplementation during pregnancy to minimize occurrence of neural tube defects
   e. Elevated levels of alpha fetoprotein **(AFP)** identified as marker for neural tube defects; presence of defect can be confirmed with ultrasound scanning techniques
   f. Significant association with development of **hydrocephalus** in association with closure of the defect and **meningitis** if closure is delayed
   g. Significant correlation with club feet and breech presentation due to fetal dyskinesia
   h. Chronic urinary tract infections due to neurologically induced bladder dysfunction

2. **Impairment:**
   a. **Cranial meningocele and Cranial encephalocele:** superior neural tube and, subsequently, cranial defects not considered spina bifida; in contrast to anencephaly, both are amenable to early surgical repair with generally optimistic outcomes
   b. **Spina Bifida Occulta:**
      - External appearance of skin over vertebral defect may be normal skin appearance, tuft of hair, dimple or sinus leading down to spinal cord
      - Typically vertebral defect only, nonfusion of vertebral arches
      - No spinal cord involvement or weakness
   c. **Spina Bifida Aperta (rachischisis or myeloschisis):**
      - Total absence of spinal cord closure
      - Appearance is often flattened plate of tissue
      - May be termed **anencephaly** if occurs at uppermost part of spinal cord resulting in minimal brain development with cerebrum typically absent
   d. **Spina Bifida Cystica:** external appearance is a fluid-filled cyst
      - **Meningocele:**
        - Cyst contains cerebrospinal fluid **(CSF)** only
        - Spinal cord remains in appropriate location
        - Little or no weakness following simple surgical repair
      - **Myelomeningocele or Meningomyelocele:**
        - Cyst contains CSF and spinal cord herniated into it
        - Depending on location and spinal cord extrusion, symptoms range from mild weakness and limited bowel and bladder incontinence to complete paraplegia, associated with hydrocephalus requiring ventriculoperitoneal shunting to drain CSF
        - Most common type of spina bifida
      - **Myelomeningocele and Hydromyelia:** same as above with addition of central canal greatly distended with CSF
   e. **Diastematomyelia:**
      - Development of two hemi spinal cords, often separated by a bony spur or block consisting of an incompletely formed vertebrae
      - May be no neurological symptoms until growth results in **tethered cord** and emergence of neurological sequelae such as rapid onset of scoliosis, lower extremity hypertonus, and urological symptoms
      - Tethered cord may occur in association with other types of spina bifida at the original surgical closure site
3. **Functional Limitations:**
   a. Highly variable depending on location and severity of spinal cord involvement
   b. Symptoms range from minimal bowel and bladder incontinence with club feet, to limited paraparesis, to complete paraplegia
   c. Weakness or absence of gluteus maximus muscles and hip adductors leading to ili-

otibial band tightness and hip flexor contractures is relatively consistent finding when generalized weakness is present, necessitating use of braces and crutches or other ambulation aids

4. **Treatment Goals and Interventions:**
   a. **Goal:** Anticipate problems and develop proactive interventions
      - With other team members, provide information to parents to promote **early identification of shunt malfunction:** increased irritability, increased muscle tone, seizures, vomiting, bulging fontanelle, headache, loss of memory, and redness along shunt tract
      - Anticipate hip flexor contractures by emphasizing full hip extension mobility at 1 year of age; minimize risk of dislocation by not forcing hip full extension before chronologically appropriate
      - Consider contribution of propped sitting to hip flexor tightness and kyphotic back alignment as child matures and evaluate whether it is an appropriate developmental skill to encourage
      - Consider allowing moderate iliotibial band tightness as means of increasing hip stability and diminishing or delaying hip subluxation or dislocation; teach caregivers not to achieve full hip adduction during range of motion activities
      - Institute standing when chronologically appropriate to encourage bone growth and increased bone density, possibly to deepen acetabulum in order to promote hip joint integrity: standing frame (Toronto A-frame), a parapodium, bilateral long leg braces, or other options

   b. **Goal:** Promote optimal trunk and extremity alignment
      - Select and teach all caregivers strategies to encourage best alignment to support typical growth and avoid or minimize contractures
      - Encourage varied sitting and standing activities with optimal trunk alignment
      - Evaluate alignment in all chairs and positional devices child uses with family, caregivers, teachers, and therapists in other environments
      - Select exercises as needed to achieve and maintain alignment

   c. **Goal:** Achieve gross, fine, and oral motor and cognitive objectives through developmental activities in younger children and functional activities in older children and adolescents
      - Whenever possible, select activities with clear functional value and measurable outcomes, rather than isolated exercises or global stimulation; evaluate on a frequent basis linkage between child's level of function and activities selected in anticipation of improvement
      - Attempt to integrate fine, gross, oral motor and cognitive objectives in multipurpose activities whenever possible

   d. **Goal:** Promote independent locomotion and independence in daily care activities
      - Encourage child's efforts at locomotion in a manner that reinforces attainment of satisfaction and promotes continued, independent efforts

- Provide assistive devices such as braces (ranging from UCB's to reciprocating gait orthoses), crutches and walkers, and wheelchairs to facilitate mobility
- Consider early selection of powered mobility devices to promote maximal environmental exploration, cognitive development, and social competence
- Promote independence in daily care activities through teamwork with child, family members, and other caregivers; select and provide assistive devices as needed to nurture independence and satisfaction in achieving it

Spinal Muscular Atrophy (see Chapter 1)

Tibial Torsion (see Table 3.1)

Torticollis (see Table 3.1)

Transient Dystonia (see Cerebral Palsy and Spastic Quadriplegia)

4 / Adaptive Equipment

Kathleen A. Harp
Andrea Santman Wiener

In addition to therapeutic handling, exercise, and functional skill training, therapeutic intervention includes maintaining biomechanical alignment, modifying the environment, and adapting activities of daily living through the use of equipment or specialized devices. The purpose of this chapter is to introduce the wide variety of equipment used with children with disabilities. Four major types of equipment will be covered: orthotics, positioning aids, mobility aids, and equipment used during treatment.

Physical therapists must consider certain factors when recommending adaptive equipment for children. These include the safety, function, maintenance, size, cost, and goal associated with using the equipment. Numerous adaptive equipment options are available to children with disabilities. To keep abreast of the most recent and appropriate equipment available, it is important for a therapist to develop a working relationship with his or her local, durable medical equipment vendor or rehabilitation technical specialist.

ORTHOTICS

Orthotics are custom made devices that assist in supporting and/or stabilizing various parts of the body to enhance functioning of those parts.

General Considerations

1. Orthotics should be designed and fabricated by individuals with experience, expertise, and specific training in pediatric biomechanics and orthotic fabrication. Children demonstrate unique biomechanical alignment; therefore, individualizing the design of an orthotic is of utmost importance.
2. Decision making should include the following:
   a. Environment in which child functions
   b. Activity level of child
   c. Musculoskeletal findings, including range of motion and joint mobility
   d. Level of caregiver's comfort in applying orthotic and monitoring skin integrity
   e. Fit of orthotic
3. Muscles controlled or supported by orthotics are not actively used by the child and therefore prone to disuse atrophy. It is important for orthotics to provide appropriate amount of support with least restrictions

Lower Extremity Orthotics

1. Purpose: to provide support to foot, ankle, knee, or hip in isolation or combination
2. General Considerations: Molded with child's foot in subtalar joint neutral position (position of foot that creates greatest congruency between talus and calcaneus)
3. Inframalleolar (IMO)
   a. Trim line inferior to malleoli
   b. Allows for movement of ankle in all planes
   c. Foot complex supported in subtalar neutral position with allowance for normal range of motion (6 °) at subtalar joint
4. Supramalleolar (SMO)
   a. Trim line superior and anterior to level of malleoli
   b. Slightly limits ankle motion and allows forward progression of tibia over foot (laterally greater than plantar flexion and dorsiflexion)
5. Ankle Foot (AFO)
   a. Crosses ankle joint and typically extends to 1/4 in below fibula head
   b. Limits plantar flexion during transitions and thus may contribute to collateral knee ligament laxity when child plays on floor
   c. Ankle set at 5–10 ° of dorsiflexion may assist in reducing genu recurvatum
      - Solid ankle; locks the ankle joint at 5–10 ° of ankle dorsiflexion
      - Articulating ankle
        - Allows movement of ankle in sagittal plane
        - Degree of plantar flexion and dorsiflexion at joint can be controlled
        - Imposes uniplanar motion on triplanar joint
      - Anterior shell
        - Molded over trim line providing an anterior segment
        - Indicated to maintain knee extension during stance
        - Full knee extension must be available passively during stance
6. Knee Ankle Foot (KAFO)
   a. Trim line is above knee
   b. Used for standing or ambulation, allowing for reciprocal or swing through gait
   c. Often used for children with spina bifida or muscular dystrophy
   d. Solid knee joint may be fixed at any appropriate angle, generally 0–5 ° of flexion
   e. Hinged knee joint allows knee to flex within a preset range of motion
   f. Various locking systems available
   g. Ankle may be solid or hinged
7. Hip Knee Ankle Foot (HKAFO) with pelvic band
   a. Extends to hip level
   b. Used for child with significant weakness in hips and lower extremities
   c. May be used bilaterally or unilaterally for ambulation; if used bilaterally, child will use swing through gait pattern
   d. Typically used for children with spina bifida or spinal cord injuries

8. Reciprocating Gait (RGO)
   a. HKAFO's with molded body jacket and cable system designed to allow for reciprocal gait; forward step is initiated with lateral weight shift
   b. Allows children with limited motor ability to ambulate and ascend stairs
   c. Used primarily for children with spina bifida or spinal cord injuries
   d. May be more energy efficient than HKAFO's
9. Isocentric Brace
   a. Similar to RGO's, but uses ball bearing system; generally easier to operate, especially for child with higher level lesion
   b. Less support given at thighs than RGO's
10. Pavlik Harness
    a. Lightweight, adjustable orthosis that places child's hips in flexion and abduction, providing greatest congruency between femoral head and acetabulum
    b. Used during the first 9 months of life for congenital hip dislocation
11. Scottish Rite Braces
    a. Provides greatest congruency between femoral head and acetabulum by placing child's hips in slight abduction with knees slightly flexed, but does not control hip rotation
    b. Has pelvic band with plastic thigh sockets
    c. Used for children >4 years of age
12. A Frame
    a. Bilateral, double upright, long leg brace with pelvic band
       - Places hips in abduction and internal rotation with knee extension and shoes wedged to keep feet in neutral
       - Metal uprights connected by horizontal bar under the groin
    b. Has length and width adjustability
    c. Used for children 9–48 months of age with congenital hip dislocation
13. Dynasplints
    a. Bracing system that provides constant tension and can be adjusted to increase range of motion
    b. Brace can be used at various joints
    c. Considerations include its high expense and complex care required

Upper Extremity Orthotics

1. Purpose:
   a. Provide support to hand, wrist, and elbow for improved function
   b. To maintain musculoskeletal alignment
2. General Considerations:
   a. Therapeutic goals should be considered when choosing splint
   b. Prefabricated splints available, but difficult to obtain good fit

   c. Children generally do not tolerate splints that make function more difficult (for example, splints that are too heavy or too restrictive likely to be unsuccessful)
   d. Splint application should be easy for parents and/or child
3. Static Splint; immobilizes the joints
   a. Spasticity reduction splint
      - Developed to reduce effects of flexor tone in hand of child with hemiplegia
      - Maintains wrist, fingers, and thumb in extension and fingers abducted
      - Splint dorsally placed on the hand
   b. Finger abduction splint; made of low temperature thermoplastic with separate holes for each finger, which maintains them in abduction and aids in extension
   c. Pneumatic splints; inflated splint that provides uniform pressure and conforms to shape of arm
4. Semidynamic splints
   a. Thumb loop
      - Loop usually made from velcro looping material which holds metacarpal of thumb in abduction
      - Assists in reducing ulnar deviation, common in children with neuromotor problems, through its attachment to wrist
      - Minimally restrictive and allows for more functional use of hand
      - Children generally tolerate well
   b. Weight bearing hand splint
      - Maintains upper extremity in position normally used in weight bearing situation
      - Used primarily during therapy to assist in developing child's ability to perform transitions
   c. Sof-splint
      - Reduces flexion and adduction of thumb
      - Easy and inexpensive to fabricate (typically made from neoprene)
      - Encourages functional use of hand
5. Dynamic Splints; have moving parts that assist in improving alignment and range of motion
   a. Orthokinetic wrist splint
      - consists of cone placed in hand that exerts pressure on wrist and hand flexors
      - forearm shell exerts pressure on forearm flexors
   b. Mackinnon splint
      - Wooden dowel placed in palm of hand to stretch intrinsic flexors; secured with strap and plastic piece on dorsum of hand
      - Fabricated for children with cerebral palsy
   c. Dynamic wrist and arch support with thumb opponens or "J splint"
      - Uses dynamic forces to maintain wrist in alignment and places pressure on hand flexors to reduce effect of flexor tone
      - Uses palmar bar that wraps around thumb in a fashion resembling letter "J"

d. Dynasplints
  - Bracing system that provides constant tension and can be adjusted to increase range of motion
  - Can be used at various joints
  - Expensive and care is complex

Spinal Orthotics

1. Purpose:
   a. Provide support to child's trunk to maintain musculoskeletal alignment
   b. Provide comfort
   c. Improve function
   d. Provide abdominal compression as one way of relieving axial loading pressure downward on spine due to gravitational load
   e. Exerts traction to align spine
2. General Considerations:
   a. Materials may need to be lighter or porous for child with respiratory compromise
   b. Used for children who lack muscular ability to hold themselves upright; provides support by circumferential pressure and stabilization of spine, minimizing extent of scoliosis development
   c. Essential to monitor skin integrity
   d. If respiratory distress present due to application of force around chest and trunk, orthotist can cut out abdominal region to allow for abdominal expansion
3. Corset
   a. Soft and prefabricated
   b. Measurements taken at waist and hips
4. Thoracolumbar Sacral Orthotic (TLSO)
   a. Soft TLSO
      - Reinforced foam material with plastic stays
      - Rigid for complete stabilization and immobilization of spine
      - Attempts to provide corrective force
      - Used for children 12–15 years of age who may develop spondylosis of 5th lumbar vertebrae
   b. Hard TLSO
      - Provides support for trunk
      - Aids in maintaining spinal alignment and may prevent increase of scoliosis

POSITIONING AIDS (Table 4.1)

Positioning aids are any pieces of equipment that promote function and assist in maintaining postural alignment to prevent musculoskeletal deformity and/or musculoskeletal limitation.

General Considerations

1. Should be monitored for safety (for example, no loose parts or sharp edges, safety belts in place, and device is stable)
2. Should be appropriate size for child
3. Alterations or modifications to piece of prefabricated equipment may negate warranty
4. Child should be monitored for signs of fatigue

Floor Based Positioners

1. Sidelyer
   a. Provides child with support in sidelying
   b. Promotes midline during functional activities; disassociation between limbs, neutral head, and trunk alignment
   c. Position child with:
      - Trunk in symmetrical position
      - Head neutral to trunk and supported
      - Weight bearing limbs slightly flexed and nonweight bearing limbs free to move
2. "Grasshopper/Tadpole" by Tumbleform
   a. Very versatile; can be used as sidelyer, prone wedge, supportive chair, or supine lyer
   b. Good option for children requiring respiratory therapy
   c. Good for center-based programs because of versatility
3. Wedge
   a. Allows child to work at an angle in supine
   b. Provides support while child is in prone
   c. Facilitates head lifting
   d. Helps position child for function
   e. Assists with postural draining in children with respiratory problems
4. Bean bags
   a. Moldable positioning device
   b. Often used for children with severe musculoskeletal deformity to support child in variety of postures
5. Boppy Support
   a. Soft "u"-shaped pillow used to help position in sitting and supine
   b. Works well with small infants
6. Rolls (half and full); used to maintain child in prone, sidelying, and sitting
7. Inner tubes
   a. Maintains hip flexion and a midline orientation with adduction of upper extremities in supine
   b. Provides support to small infant in sitting by providing boundaries on all sides

8. Sand bags; used for support
9. Knee skis (Figure 4.1)
   a. Provide support in kneeling position
   b. Prevent child from "W"-sitting and excessive hip abduction
   c. Caregivers should monitor lower extremity skin integrity

Standing Devices (Figures 4.2 and 4.3)

1. Purpose:
   a. Promotes weight bearing through lower extremities for prevention of bone demineralization
   b. Allows face-to-face interaction with peers and adults
2. Prone stander
   a. Used to gain physiological benefits from weight bearing
   b. Total support to anterior part of body
   c. Position angle from upright can be varied to provide:
      - Varying amounts of head control
      - Differing/varying amounts of weight bearing of both upper and lower extremities
      - Varying tray positions

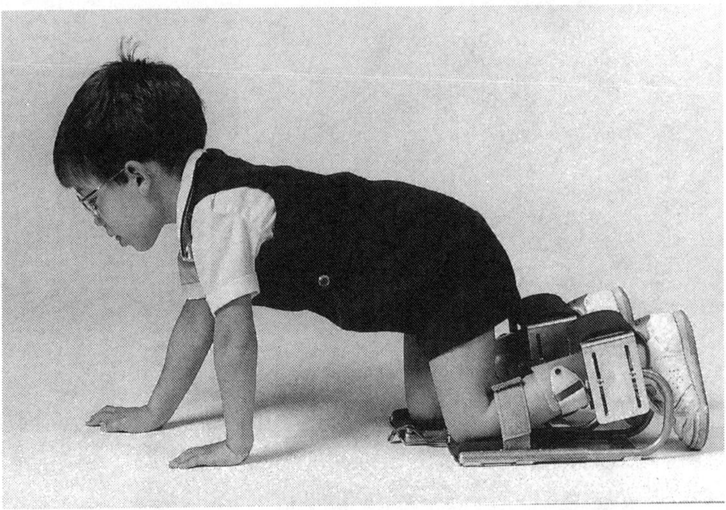

Figure 4.1. Knee skis.

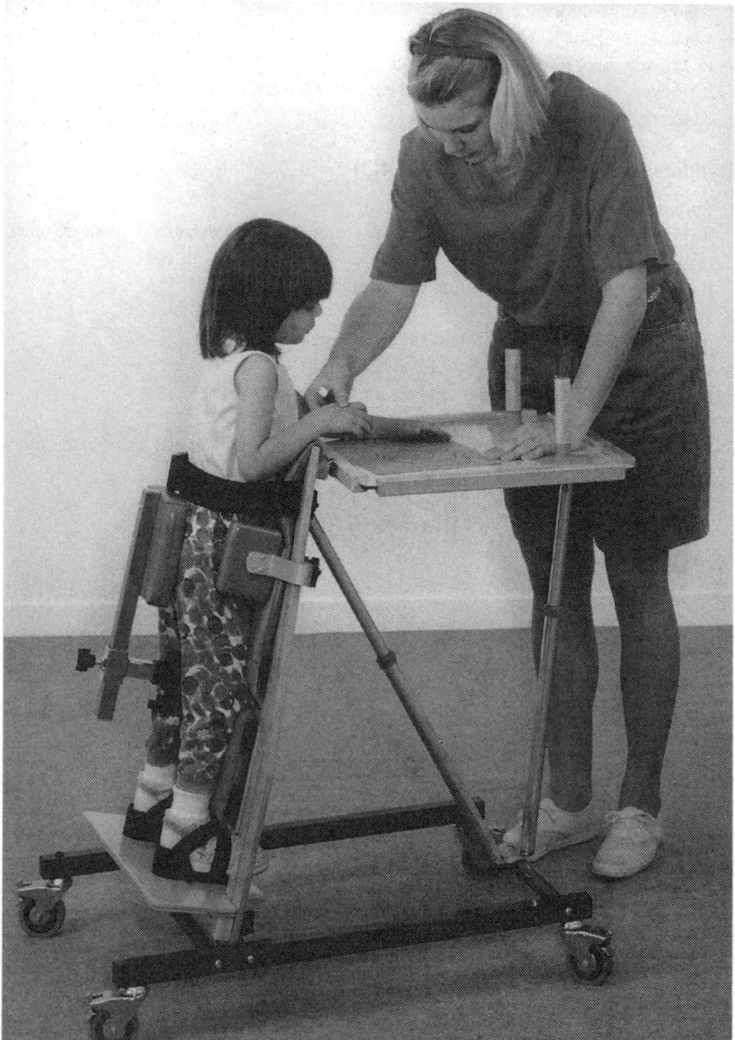

Figure 4.2. Prone stander.

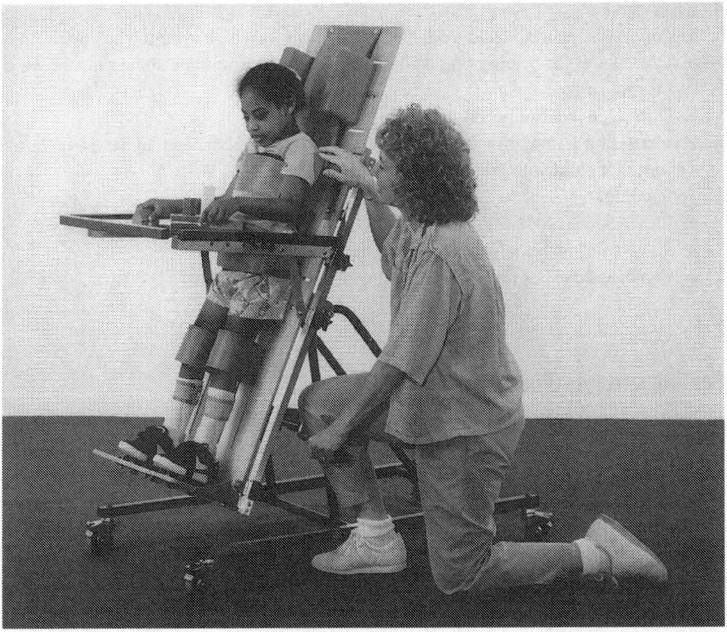

Figure 4.3. Supine stander.

   d. Wheels make it easily transportable to increase opportunity for interaction with peers and family; allows increased mobility
3. Standing box
   a. 4-sided box system with tray
   b. Difficult to position child properly
4. Supine stander
   a. Support to posterior surface of body
   b. Can be placed in various angles from vertical to horizontal to adjust for amount of head control and weight bearing through lower extremities; does not provide weight bearing through upper extremities
   c. Fact that supine stander is large piece of equipment should be considered when choosing this piece of equipment

5. Knee stander
   a. Provides support to child's pelvis and trunk while in high kneeling position
   b. Child's weight bearing on patella is cause of concern; knee should not be weight bearing surface
   c. Difficult to control pelvis
6. Free standing frame: provides support through trunk, pelvis, and leg straps in vertical standing for child with greater trunk control
7. Parapodium
   a. Provides total contact and support at child's ankles, knees, hips, and trunk
   b. Allows for mobility by using swivel motion
   c. Can be used as 1st orthosis for child with neural tube defect

Seating systems (Figures 4.4 and 4.5)

Prescribing seating systems for the pediatric population can be quite complex. Frequently, a seating system is recommended that is to be placed in a wheeled mobility system. It is important to remember for documentation purposes that the seating system is separate from the wheeled mobility base or wheelchair.

Seating systems can also be stable, stand alone devices. These are most often prefabricated systems with limited adjustability and options.

Careful consideration of necessary supports is important for the pediatric population. Children with neuromotor problems are typically at risk for musculoskeletal deformity such as contractures and scoliosis. For instance, children with cerebral palsy often have a tendency to push into extension, which may be decreased by making the hip angle more acute. In addition, because children's bodies are growing and changing rapidly, the ability of seating systems to "grow" is a primary consideration.

1. Purpose: to provide optimal postural alignment for functional activities including mobility and activities of daily living
2. General Considerations
   a. Pelvic positioning straps should be provided with all seating systems; essential that pelvis be positioned in stable manner with pelvic positioning strap placed over iliac crest
   b. Seat and foot angles should be determined based on each individual's functional goals
   c. Seating systems should be monitored for safety (for example, no loose parts or sharp edges, safety belts in place, and device is stable)
   d. System must be appropriate size for child
   e. If therapist alters or modifies prefabricated seating system, then warranty may be negated

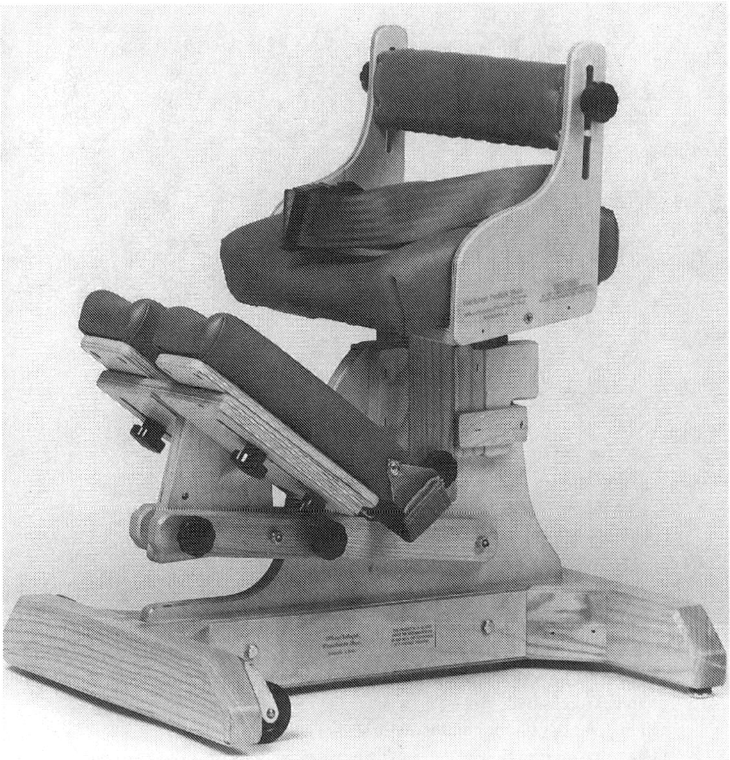

Figure 4.4. Posture chair.

f. In designing seating system:
- Parameters of seat height and depth, back, arm rests, and seat to back angle should be taken into consideration
- Consideration and guidelines established for adults should generally be followed
- The following are particular to pediatric population:
  - Seat width - 1" on each side
  - Seat depth - consider energy-efficient alignment for propulsion when adding cushioning to decrease seat depth
  - Back rest height- consider head rest/head support system

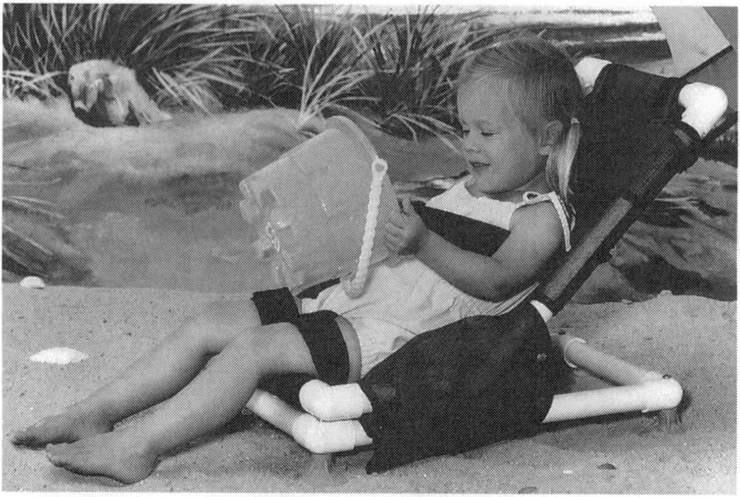

Figure 4.5. Shower or bath chair.

3. Custom Seating Systems
   a. Molded (contoured positioning insert (CPI) and contour U system by Pindot)
      - Custom fit provides intimate contact between child and seat distributing biomechanical forces over greater area
      - Often good option for children with severe spinal deformities
      - Generally used with wheeled mobility base but significantly increases weight of wheelchair and makes folding of the chair more difficult
   b. Linear seating systems
      - Uses planar supports in configuration to support child in good postural alignment; configuration based on individual needs of child
      - Less expensive than molded seats and provides more room for growth
4. Options available; same for adults and children; below are listed some of more commonly used options with pediatric population
   a. Lateral trunk supports
      - Promotes trunk symmetry
      - Proper placement of support essential in promoting optimal alignment and prevention of skin breakdown

b. Medial thigh support
  - Assists in maintaining hips in neutral for children who tend to hold lower extremities in adduction
  - Ensure placement which is sufficiently anterior, as this should not be used as anti-slip wedge or crotch support
  - Wedge needs to cover wide area to avoid skin breakdown
  - Must be used with pelvic positioning strap
c. Lateral thigh support
  - Assists in maintaining legs in neutral for child who tends to keep legs in abduction
  - Proper placement of support essential to maintain optimal hip alignment
d. Head supports
  - Prior to providing head support, pelvis, trunk, and shoulders should be well supported in optimum position
  - Provides support for child who has difficulty with head control
  - Various amounts of support provided by different head rests
  - May be necessary during transport even for child with fairly good head control
  - May be lateral or posterior; in some cases anterior head band may be used, but most children with significant lack of head control need combination of lateral and posterior support
  - Henslinger; provides maximal support around neck to prevent head movement in any direction
e. Reverse wedges; create more acute angle at hip joint to decrease tendency of pushing into extension
f. Cushion
  - Generally made of soft dense material to prevent skin breakdown and increase child's comfort
  - Changes back height and arm rest height; lowers foot plate in relation to child, thus should consider when measuring
g. Upper extremity support tray
  - Tray is either wood or clear plexiglas
  - Used for upper extremity support
  - Useful for mounting of computers or communication devices
h. Anterior trunk supports
  - Shoulder straps should be inserted at shoulder level or slightly below and pulled down behind child to promote shoulder depression, retraction, and placement of head in midline upright position
  - "H" harness: frontal support with straps going up and over shoulders and one across the pelvis; bottom strap of "H" harness should not be attached to seat belt

- Shoulder retractors: apparatus attached to seating system that comes anterior to shoulder girdle in order to assist in maintaining shoulder depression and more erect posture in seating system

5. Prefabricated Seating Systems
   a. Snug seat; removable foam inserts allowing customized fit and security
   b. Trip Trapp
      - Wooden seat that adjusts at seat depth, back support height, and foot rest level
      - Easily placed under conventional table
      - Safety belt (pelvic strap) and/or arm rests may or may not be present
   c. Corner seat
      - Assists in keeping shoulder girdle forward and head in midline
      - Places hips at 90 ° angle to trunk
      - Can be placed flat on floor or raised up on platform
   d. Bolster seat
      - Maintains lower extremities in abduction
      - Child may compensate by holding legs in adduction against bolster
   e. "Carrie Seat" by Tumbleform
      - Soft, plastic molded seating system with footrests, headrests, and adjustable tray
      - Difficult to place child's pelvis in neutral position because of roundness of lumbar region
   f. "Feeder Chair" by Tumbleform
      - Molded plastic seating system which can be placed on floor
      - Places pelvis in posterior pelvic tilt and biases entire spine towards flexion
      - Rarely places child in functional position due to bias toward flexion and angle of seat
   g. Kinder Chair
      - Provides support for better trunk and head control
      - Places hips, knees, and ankles at 90 °
   h. Computer ergonomic chair; provides child seating position which places pelvis in anterior pelvic tilt which, in turn, promotes spinal extension and good neck and head alignment
   i. Posture Chair by TheraAdapt (Figure 4.4)
      - Similar to computer chair but allows more adjustability
      - Supports for trunk and head control
      - Places hips, knees, and ankles at 90 °
      - May cause increased lordosis in child with excessive anterior pelvic tilt
   j. Shower and bath chairs (Figure 4.5)
      - Provides postural support, alignment, and safety while bathing
      - Especially useful for children and adolescents with severe musculoskeletal involvement

k. Cube chair
    - Provides minimal support for better trunk and head control
    - Provides minimal support for hips, knees, and ankles at 90 °

MOBILITY AIDS

Mobility aids include those devices which assist in seated or standing mobility as well as those which assist with ambulation.

Purpose:

Mobility aids provide options for mobility while maintaining optimal postural alignment for functional activities.

General Considerations

1. Should be monitored for safety (for example, no loose parts or sharp edges, device is stable, tires properly maintained, and wheel locks functional)
2. System must be appropriate size for child
3. If therapist alters or modifies prefabricated mobility aide, alteration may negate warranty
4. Type of seating system to be used with wheeled mobility base must fit child appropriately and accommodate needs of child and family
5. Mobility base should be chosen after determining positioning needs and fitting of seating system
6. Often children with neuromotor problems need a special adaptation, such as tilt in space, to assist with prevention of reflux or to minimize fatigue
7. Parents of young children often find stroller type bases more acceptable and easier to maneuver

Wheeled Mobility Bases

1. Manual wheelchair
    a. Chair propelled by upper extremities
    b. Less expensive option
2. Manual one arm drive
    a. Wheelchair can be driven with one arm; both hand wheel controls on one side
    b. Older model's frame not as stable
3. Stroller bases
    a. Typically have 4 relatively small wheels and resemble baby strollers
    b. Child using this type of base dependent on others for mobility
    c. Mounting seating systems on these bases can be difficult and require extra mounting hardware

Table 4.1. Problem Solving Considerations for Seating Systems

Problem	Neuromotor	Orthopedic	Functional/ Environmental	Evaluation	Possible Solutions
I. Pelvis a. Posterior tilt (sacral sitting—no lumbar curve)	Central hypotonia Bias toward flexion	Tight hamstrings combined with: Seat too long Anterior wedge too high Footrests too low Limited hip flexion	Not seated far enough back in seat due to improper placement Seat belt too high (above ASIS)	Determine appropriate orientation in space Review degree of hamstring tightness	Add knee block to maintain neutral pelvic alignment if posture is not fixed Tilt system back to decrease gravity's effect on spine Use lumbar/sacral pad Alter position of head relative to position in space Shorten seat depth, allowing knees to come under, if necessary; custom footrests to allow knees to flex Decrease amount of wedging Reposition pelvis, reinforce instructions to caregivers Reposition lap belt

Table 4.1. continued

Problem	Neuromotor	Orthopedic	Functional/ Environmental	Evaluation	Possible Solutions
b. Lateral tilt	Asymmetry of muscle tone	Scoliosis Subluxation/ dislocation of hip	Sling seat of wheelchair Seat too narrow	Evaluate flexibility of pelvis for possible realignment Review seating surface Review abnormal pathology Review for development of scoliosis/dislocated hip	Solid seat with lateral pelvic blocks for midline orientation Build up under buttock-low side if deformity is flexible, high side if deformity is fixed
c. Pelvic rotation	Asymmetry of muscle tone Limited variety of movement patterns available	Scoliosis with rotational component Thigh length discrepancy Subluxation/ dislocation of hip	Fit seat of chair for thigh which is apparently longer	Check to see whether scoliosis is fixed or flexible Assess muscle tone and biomechanical/musculoskeletal alignment	Midline positioning of head to reduce effects of asymmetry Midline, firm pelvic positioning If fixed deformity, allow pelvis and lower extremities to rotate and to achieve forward position of head and trunk With thigh length discrepancy, accommodate leg lengths individually

Table 4.1. continued

Problem	Neuromotor	Orthopedic	Functional/ Environmental	Evaluation	Possible Solutions
II. Hips a. Extension/ adduction	Increased bias toward extension	Dislocation of hip(s)	Seat too short, causing inadequate pelvic/thigh support Hammocking of seat Insufficient hip flexion to overcome extensor tone	Check whether hip flexion results in adequate relaxation of adductors (may not be possible to gain correction with hip dislocation) Review position of body in space	Seat depth 1½" shorter than "back of buttock to knee crease" measurement Anterior wedge (usually 10–15° with firm base) (hip flexion can facilitate abduction/external rotation pattern) increase wedge depth only if no other way to control. With deeper wedges, watch length of sitting period in relation to circulation (compression on blood flow at hip/knee) Remove footrest temporarily if necessary Pommel—distal ⅓ of medial thigh

Table 4.1. continued

Problem	Neuromotor	Orthopedic	Functional/ Environmental	Evaluation	Possible Solutions
b. Flexion/ abduction	Hypotonic/ athetoid Flexion/adduction, internal rotation pattern	Surgical adductor release		Review position of head in space	Ensure that head is in neutral orientation Lateral thigh blocks maintain neutrality with adequate stable base for sitting (30–40° abduction) Change functional work to eye level as much as possible
c. Internal/external rotation	Abnormal tone	Surgical abductor release	May be stimulated by poor positioning of pelvis in seat Sling seat Improper pommel position combined with poor foot position	If abduction/adduction problems are corrected adequately, this should provide control needed	Internal rotation—lateral extensions can be placed on footrest Soft leg ties can sometimes be used (avoid if possible) Neutral foot positioning often must block both laterally and medially to alleviate internal rotation posturing

4. Hemi chairs
    a. Frame placed lower to ground so child may propel him or herself with lower extremities
    b. Height from floor may place young child closer to level of peers
5. Power mobility systems

Power mobility systems are motorized wheelchairs. They provide a more energy efficient means of mobility for children that have difficulty self propelling a manual wheelchair; they also increase a child's sense of environmental control and independence and allow the child to keep up with his or her peers.

Some considerations include: they are heavier and require more care (for example, the battery needs to be charged routinely), they require a functional control mechanism, and they require an 18–24 month cognitive level (minimum) to learn control of the mobility device.

   a. Add on
      - Motorized component that converts a manual chair to power system
      - Not good on all terrains due to lack of frame stability
   b. Modular base
      - Powered system with 4 small wheels; heavy and sits low to ground
      - Good for varied terrain
      - Accommodates any type of seating system including reclining and tilt in space
      - Limited portability due to weight of chair
   c. Standard
      - Powered system with large rear wheels
      - Good for indoor and outdoor terrain
      - Can accommodate any type of seating system or control mechanism
      - Limited portability
   d. Scooters/Three Wheelers (for example, Pony and Amigos)
      - Powered mobility with seat that rotates to side for easy transfers in and out of chair; handlebars mounted on central tiller
      - Good for children; however, they must have adequate sitting balance due to limited postural support
      - Large turning radius
      - Child needs enough upper extremity control to move handlebars

6. Wheelchair Options

Generally all the options available to the adult are available to children. Considerations when choosing wheelchair options for adults are similar to choosing those appropriate for children. The following will discuss only those considerations unique to children to assist in decision making. Those options discussed under section, Seating Systems; are appropriate to consider in designing a power mobility system.

a. Frame options
   - Solid; lighter weight frame for wheelchair
   - Folding (collapsible)
     - Wheel base that folds is more convenient for stowing and transporting; however, folding frame may not be as stable on variety of different terrains

b. Footrests
   - Provides support for lower extremities when child is seated in seating system
   - Elevating footrests; add significantly to weight of wheelchair
   - Swing away footrests

c. Toe and heel loops
   - Maintains foot securely on footrest, preventing foot from sliding behind or in front of foot plate
   - Often necessary for children with neuromotor problems such as cerebral palsy

d. Brakes (wheel locks) handle extension provides greater lever arm, making it easier for child to engage or disengage wheel lock

e. Grade aids prevent chair from rolling backward when child is propelling wheelchair uphill

f. Quick release wheels allow easier transporting of wheelchair in smaller compartment (for example, a car trunk)

g. Wheel grips can be placed horizontal, vertical, or at diagonal on hand rim to allow for improved ease of propelling

h. Power control mechanisms
   - Variety of options available; selection should consider body parts that provide accurate, reliable, energy efficient movements
   - Hand control joy stick is mechanism of choice (proportional drive or micro switch)
   - Position joystick most functional for child, often at midline for child with neuromotor problems

7. Travel chair (Mulholland, Orthokinetic, Safety Travel)
   a. Seating system with wheeled base in which child can be transported safely in standard 4-door car
   b. Very complex to assemble and dismantle; some very adaptable

Ambulation Aids

1. Assists child to maintain balance or give lateral support during upright forward progression
2. General Considerations
   a. Environment in which child is to function should be considered when choosing ambulation aide; for example, steps may make crutches better option than walker

b. Children often in transition between different kinds of aids and therefore may need more than one option available to them on regular basis
c. Initially height of ambulation device can be traditionally placed slightly higher to promote erect standing

3. Walkers
   a. Wide base of support
   b. Support taken through upper extremities
   c. Heavier walkers may add stability for children with ataxia
   d. Children with significant muscle weakness may benefit from walker with fewer adaptations to decrease weight
   e. Forward walker
      - Walker that provides support from front
      - Encourages trunk flexion during ambulation; can be excessive and lead to increased crouch gait pattern
      - Encourages pushing through upper extremities
   f. Posterior walker (postural control walker) (Figure 4.6)
      - Provides support from rear
      - Often recommended to increase trunk extension
      - Encourages upper extremity position of shoulder depression and extension, elbow extension, and neutral wrist
      - Children may tend to sit back on horizontal crossbar of walker; bungee cord placed across rear of walker may help to prevent this
   g. Ring walkers
      - Provide support around trunk and under crotch
         - Children often sit on strap and propel themselves with bent legs
         - If more independent ambulation is goal, this does not develop good lower extremity strength and coordination for upright mobility
      - Wheeled base
      - Large base of support precludes from being functional option for most children
   h. Gait trainer (Figure 4.7)
      - Significant support provided to upper extremities and trunk
      - Allows child with severe motor impairments to propel self with lower extremities
      - Expensive
      - Manufacturer advocates supervision of child at all times
   i. Walker options
      - Arm rests
         - Support forearm and hand
         - Attach to walker base

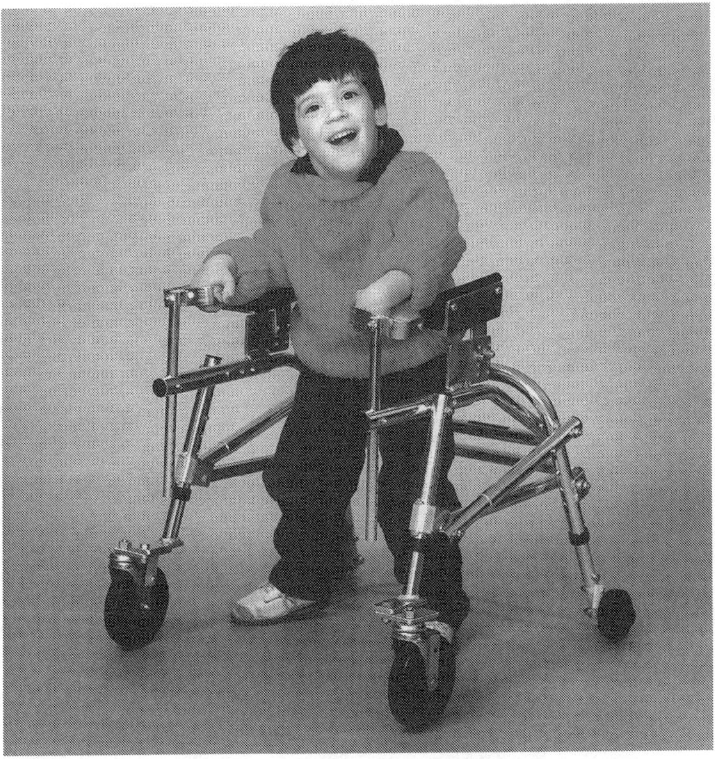

Figure 4.6. Postural control walker.

- Extra long base
  - Provides wider anterior posterior base of support, making it less likely to tip
  - Children learning to use RGO's often start with this type of walker
- Grade aids; prevent rollator walker from going backwards down an incline
- Wheels
  - Forward or posture control walker with wheels is rollator walker
  - Wheels can be placed on 2–4 legs of walker

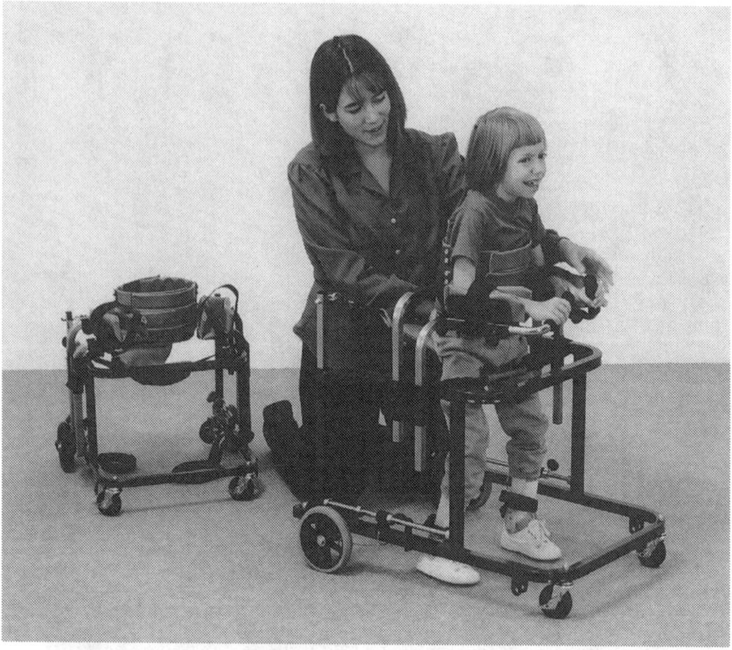

Figure 4.7. Gait trainer.

- ◦ Does not require child to lift up walker to propel self forward
- ◦ Swivel wheels allow for easier turning, but more difficult to control

4. Crutches
   a. General Considerations:
      - Crutches require child to have greater postural control than walkers
      - As with adults, axillary or loftstrand crutches are available
   b. Crutch options
      - Large crutch tip
        - ◦ Large rubber tip substitutes for standard tip, providing more stable contact between crutch and floor
        - ◦ Large crutch tips good option for children with new crutches

- Forearm supports
    - Provide support from elbow to hand and holds elbow at approximately 90 ° for greater weight bearing surface
    - Make crutches an option for children with limited hand and arm function
    - Increase weight of crutches

5. Canes; types and fitting are same as for adult population

TREATMENT EQUIPMENT

Treatment equipment assists the therapist during treatment. The equipment may provide biomechanical support, assisting the therapist and child in controlling movement. Use of treatment equipment also helps to encourage active participation of the child during therapy. Finally, treatment equipment helps to provide a variety of options to the therapist and child toward achieving functional goals.

General Considerations

1. Be aware of safety
2. Maintain variety to interest the child
3. Other people (parents, teachers, and/or direct care providers) must be trained in appropriate, safe use of equipment and precautions to be aware of during equipment use
4. All equipment (especially mobile surfaces) requires practice by therapist to control surface and to handle child

Ball/ Bolsters/ Rolls

1. Provides moving surface to facilitate postural adjustments and balance reactions
2. Depending on speed of movement, can be relaxing or stimulating
3. Consider properties when treatment planning (sizes, colors, textures, and shape); all properties may affect child's interest, enjoyment, and treatment success
4. Bolsters can be used for positioning, dynamic sitting activities, lateral balance activities, or range of motion activities, including runners lunge

Bench

1. Adjustable height; used to facilitate cruising and transitions (floor to sit and sit to stand)
2. Dynamic bench, "Theradapt"
    a. On rocking legs to provide mobile treatment surface
    b. Assists in encouraging equilibrium reaction

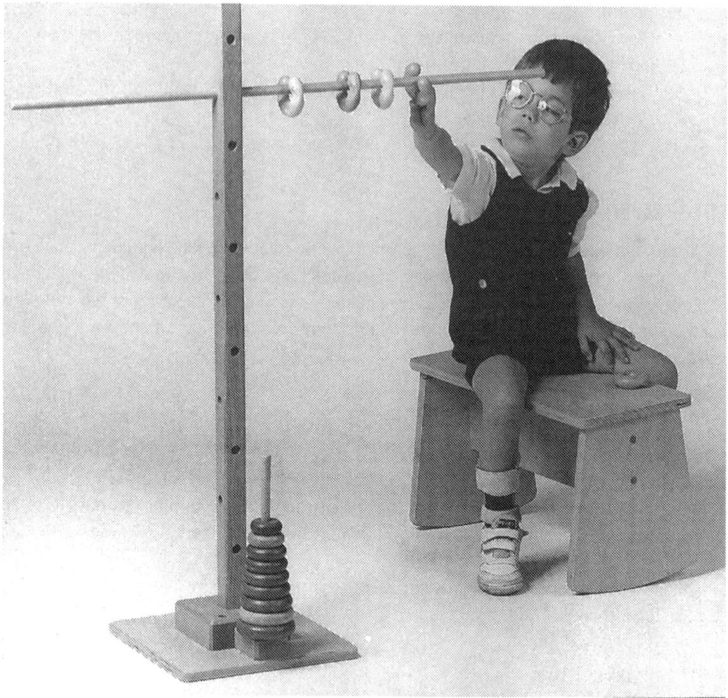

Figure 4.8. Bench.

Crawler

Provides support to child's trunk in quadruped, facilitating forward propulsion

Educubes

1. Chairs which are not supportive or adjustable
2. Adaptable to 2 seating levels
3. Can be used as table

Scooterboard

1. Wooden, plastic, or carpet-covered base with 4 wheels; similar to flat skateboard, allowing prone mobility
2. Used to increase upper extremity extensor strength, shoulder forward flexion, thoracic extension, head lifting, and sensory feedback
3. Various sizes and shapes

Standing poles

1. 2 vertical poles that child holds onto to promote upright posture and balance
2. May be used to initiate ambulation

"T" stools

Chair with one leg to challenge child's sitting balance

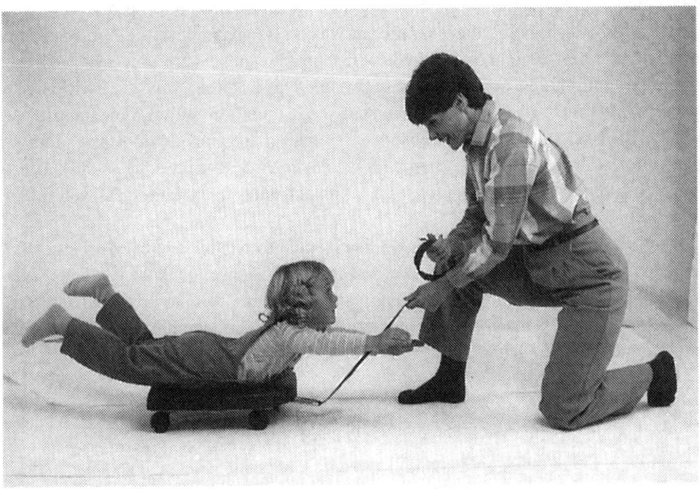

Figure 4.9. Scooterboard.

Tilt Board (equilibrium reactions)

Provides mobile surface for child to respond adaptively to displacement

"Ready Racer Tumbleforms"

1. Toy car made of soft foam with pneumatic tires so that child can sit in and be low to ground and propel themselves
2. A pre wheelchair device

Dycem

1. Piece of rubberized plastic that can be placed under equipment to prevent equipment from sliding
2. Good to put under plates to prevent sliding while child is eating
3. Can place on seat to prevent slippage

Sensory Integration Equipment (see Table 4.2)

Sensory integration is based on three basic principles. First, typical individuals are able to receive information from their bodies and the environment, process and interpret the information within their central nervous systems, and use the information in a functional manner. Second, individuals with problems in sensory processing will have problems planning and performing motor acts. Third, if the individual with sensory processing dysfunction is provided the sensory stimulation within a meaningful context, he or she will integrate the sensory information and thus demonstrate more efficient motor skills and adaptive behaviors. Sensory integration equipment is used to engage children actively in sensory stimulation activities in a meaningful, self directed context.

When planning a treatment session, it is essential to provide a safe environment. The equipment can be very mobile, unstable, and fast to challenge the child's various sensory systems. During treatment, it is important to encourage the child to be as active as possible. Table 4.2 outlines the goals of treatment and the types of equipment used to assist the child in obtaining therapeutic goals.

Table 4.2. Uses of Sensory Integration Equipment

Goal	Equipment	Description
Promoting antigravity flexion	Bolster swing	Encourages antigravity flexion or postural balance in sitting
	Flexion disc/yellow and blue flexion swing	Swing with flat disc and center post at right angles to each other Holding center post develops flexion muscles Varying degrees of difficulty based on amount of support from flexion swing
	Rope ladder	Suspended from ceiling; used to encourage motor planning and improve strength and eye-foot coordination
	Trapeze bar swing	
	Zip swing or flying trapeze	Horizontal glider; also used to increase tolerance to movement
	Inner tube	
	Hot dog swing	Vertical bolster
Promoting thoracic extension	Hammock swing (sling swing)	Provides support to child in prone to encourage head and thoracic extension
	Scooterboard	Wooden, plastic, or carpet-covered base with 4 wheels; similar to flat skateboard allowing prone mobility; various sizes and shapes Also used to increase upper extremity extensor strength, shoulder forward flexion, head lifting, thoracic extension, and sensory feedback
	Barrel	Lying prone over barrel, child walks his or her hands forward to encourage thoracic extension

Table 4.2. continued

Goal	Equipment	Description
Promoting gravitational security	Cocoon swing Hammock swing Platform swing Trampoline/bouncing pad	Provides graded movement experiences controlled by child to gradually increase tolerance to movement
Promoting balance and equilibrium	Bolster swing	Encourages antigravity flexion or postural balance in sitting
	Hippity-hop ball	Ball with handle that child sits on top of and bounces to move it forward
	Platform swing	Large, flat, square surface providing therapist large, mobile surface to challenge child's balance and equilibrium reactions
	T-stool	Small disc with short vertical pole; child sits on it and maintains balance; incorporates upper extremity activities while sitting
Promoting proprioceptive feedback	Hippity-hop ball	
	Weighted vests and collars	Advantageous for children with ataxia
Provide vestibular stimulation	Scooterboard	
	Sit and Spin	Commercially available flat disc that child sits on and turns him or herself in circles by turning a center wheel Provides vestibular stimulation and increased flexor strength
	Trampoline Bolster swing Foam blocks and crash pad (moon pad) Hammock swing	
Promoting motor planning	Rope ladder Barrel	

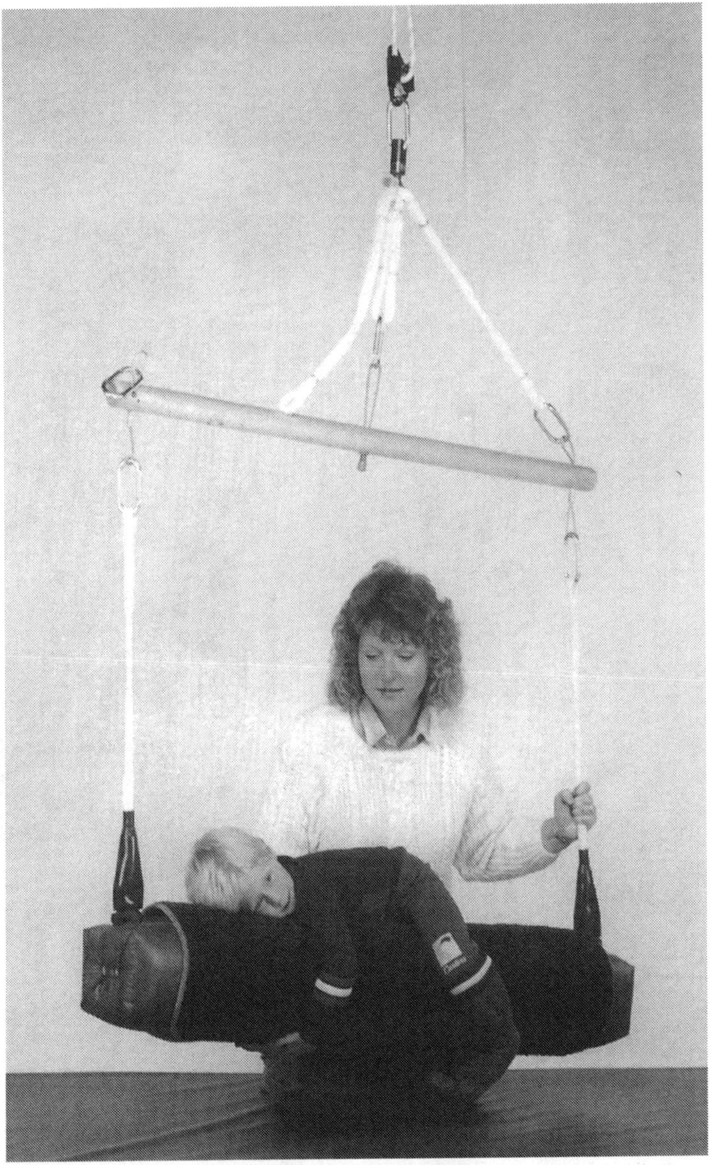

Figure 4.10. Bolster swing.

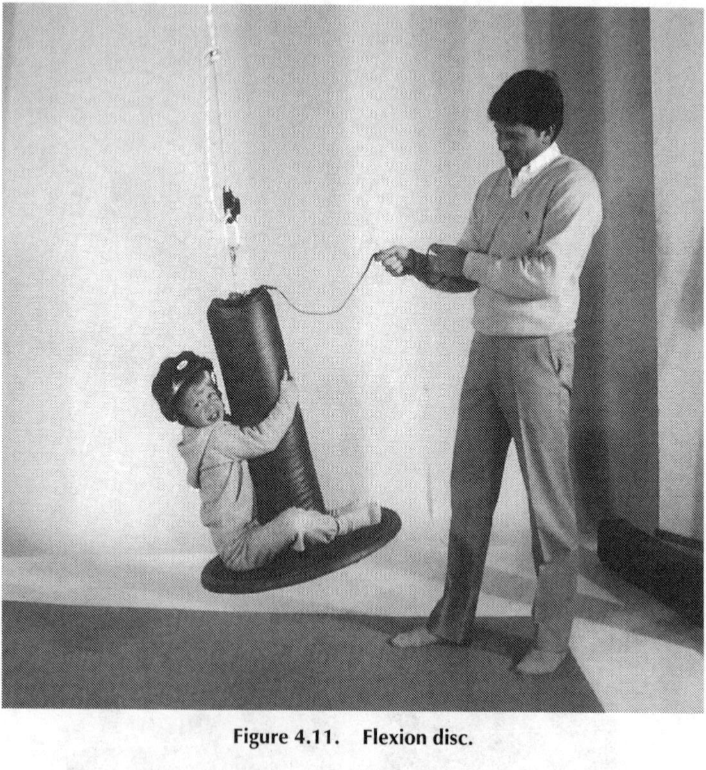

Figure 4.11. Flexion disc.

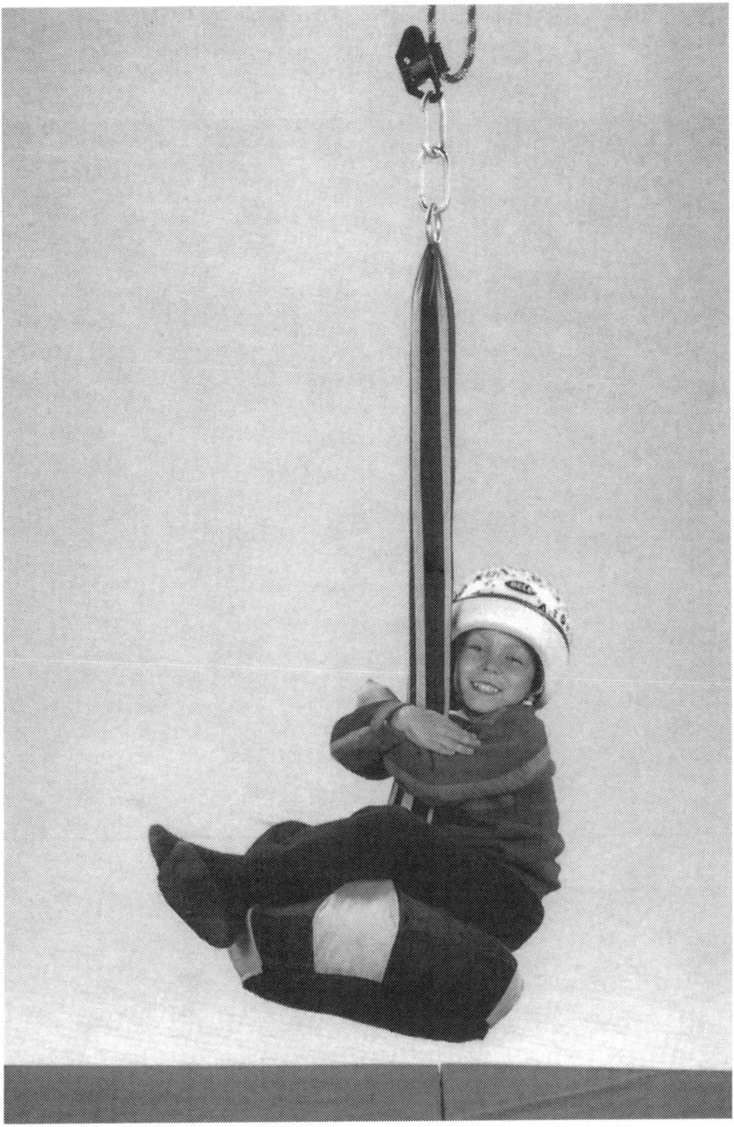

Figure 4.12. Flexion swing.

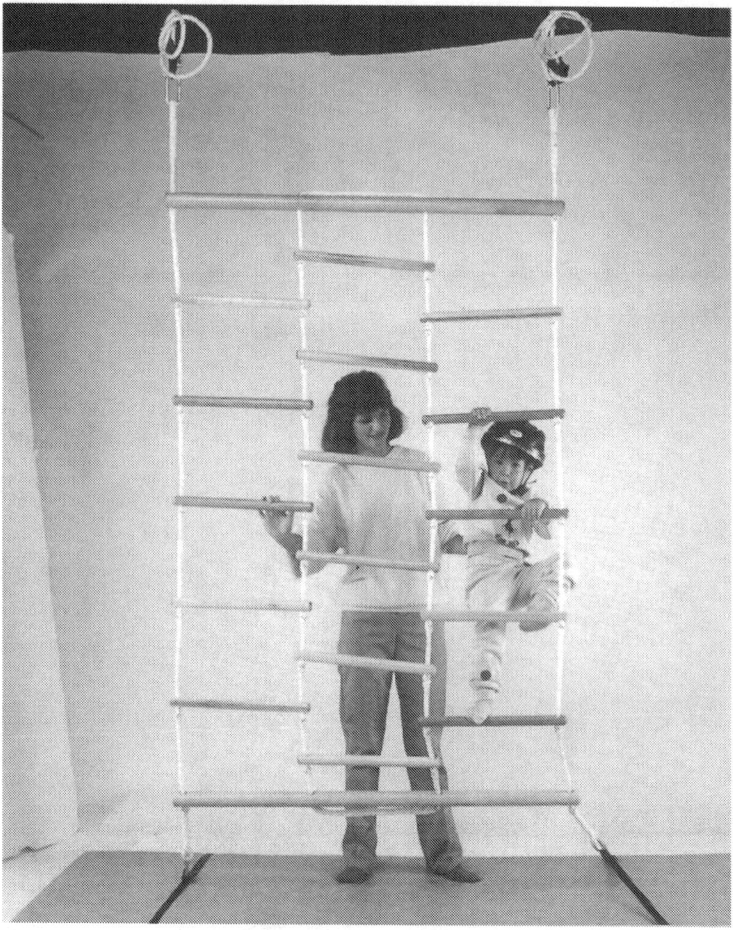

Figure 4.13. Rope ladder.

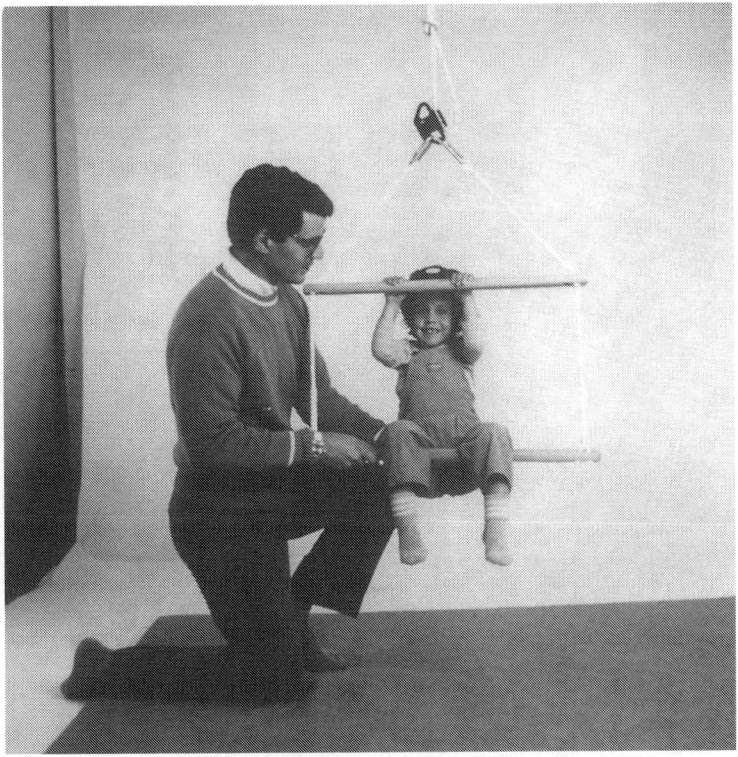

Figure 4.14. Trapeze bar swing.

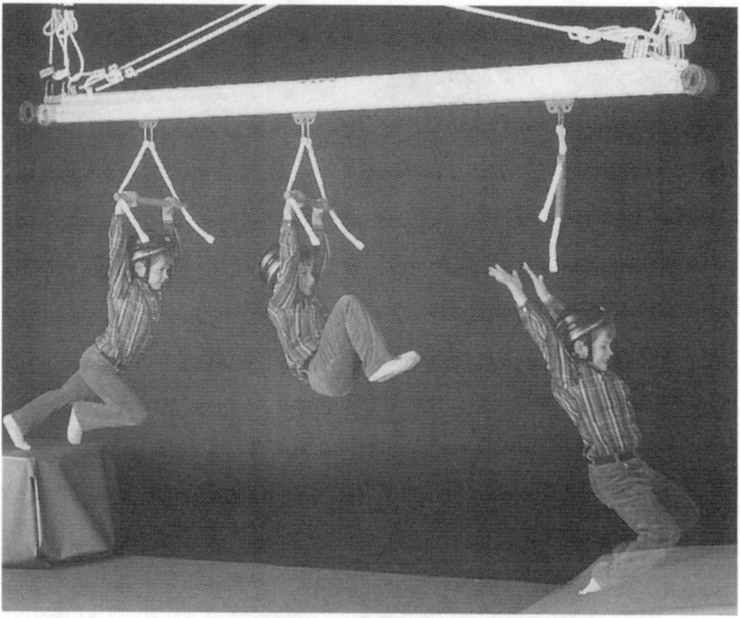

Figure 4.15. Zip swing flying trapeze.

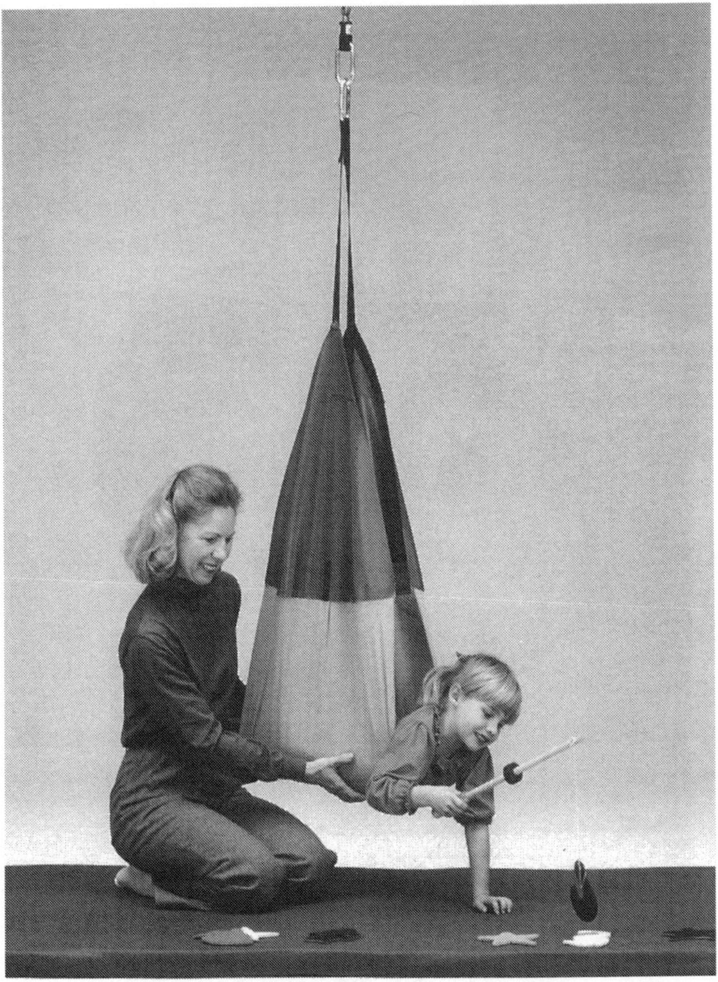

Figure 4.16. Hammock swing/slide swing.

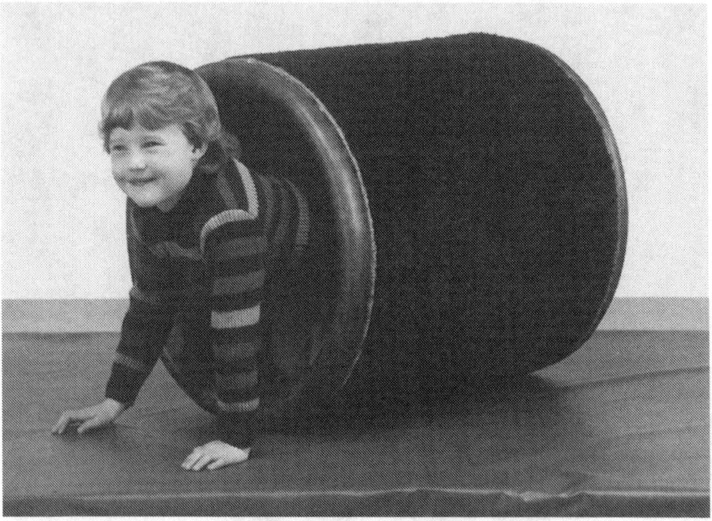

Figure 4.17. Barrel.

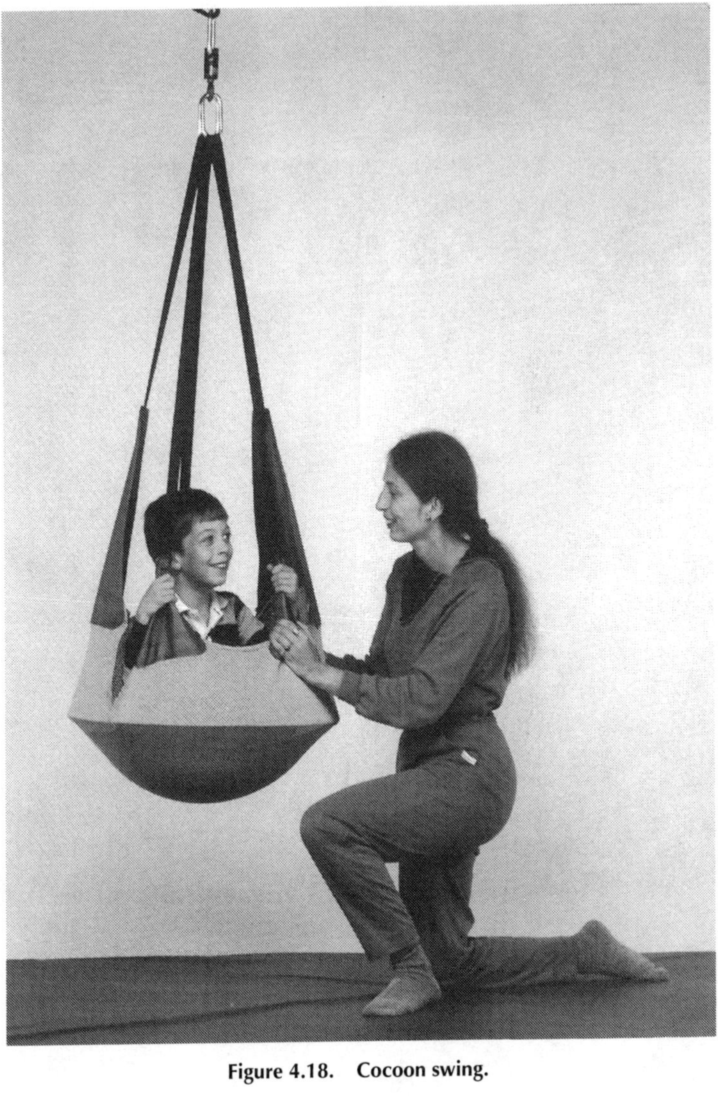

Figure 4.18. Cocoon swing.

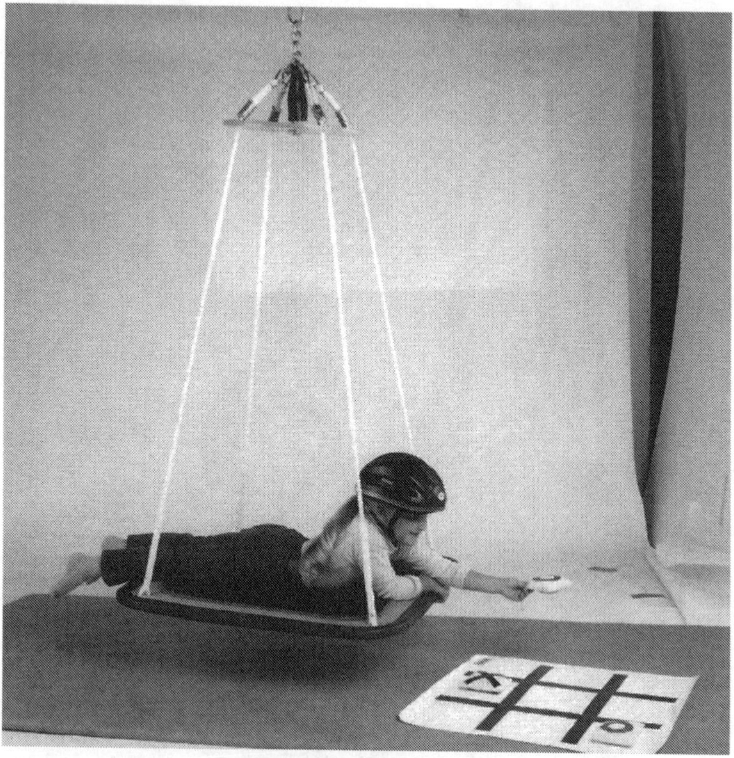

Figure 4.19. Platform swing.

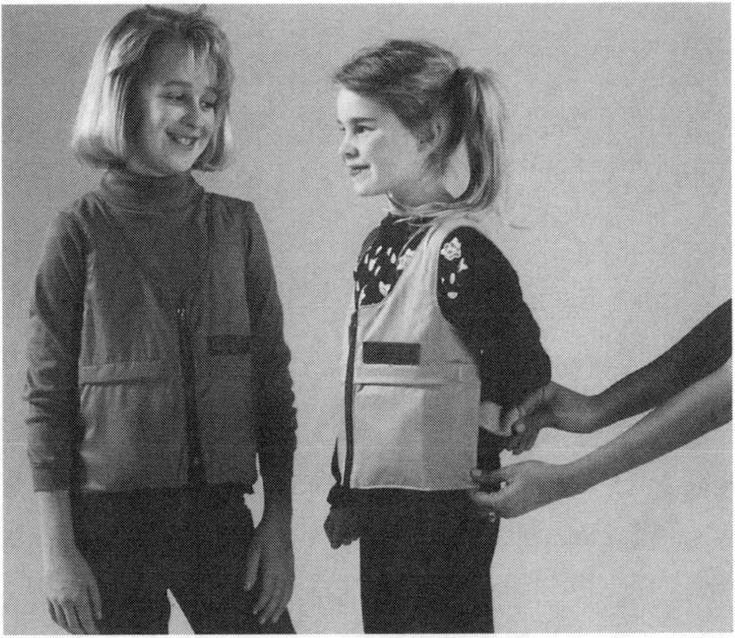

Figure 4.20. Weighted vests.

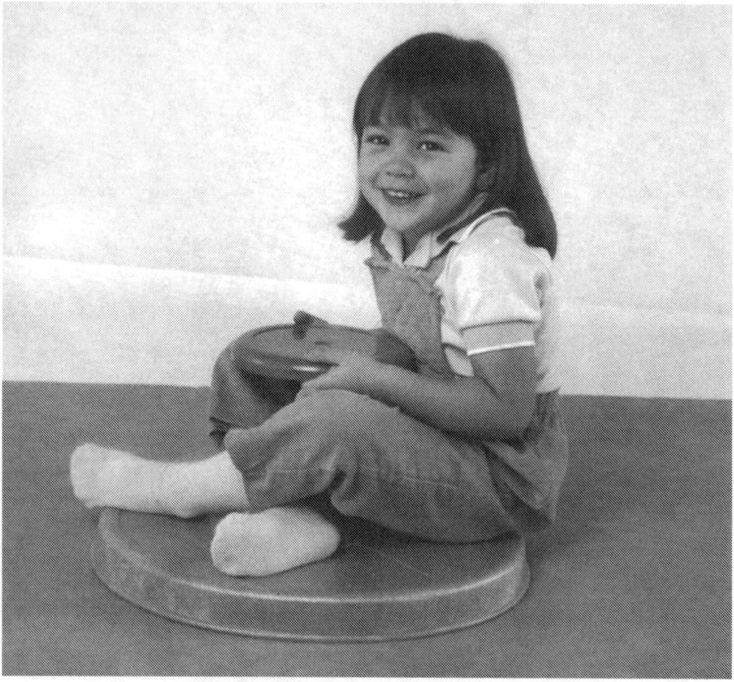

Figure 4.21. Sit and spin.

5 / Locomotion

Holly Lea Cintas

Movement occurring in the context of human locomotion is characterized by fluidity, reciprocation, and symmetry, whether related to the task of walking or to the optimal performance of a ballerina or an ultra athlete. The beauty of average or abnormally superior locomotor capability may be unappreciated unless contrasted with a movement disorder.

Children with locomotor disorders represent a large proportion of the population of children treated by pediatric physical therapists. Their resource needs may be significant until the locomotor problem is resolved or compensated. At the same time, the plasticity present during the first 5 years of locomotor maturation, and the availability of remaining growth, are windows of opportunity for timely and effective physical therapy intervention.

PRENATAL LOCOMOTION (SEE TABLE 5.1)

Prenatal locomotion repositions the fetus within the uterus and is critical for joint development. From 10–16 weeks' gestational age (GA), rotation of the fetal body relative to the axis of the umbilical cord, assisted by leg push-offs, is a typical form of locomotor behavior. Creeping or climbing efforts against the uterine wall occur by 14–15 weeks. By 17–18 weeks' GA, vigorous lower extremity thrusts off the uterine wall which incorporate full hip extension are well established. With continuing growth and uterine confinement, these thrusts become the primary form of locomotion, probably contributing to the fetal ability to position the head in the birth canal.

NEONATAL LOCOMOTION

Very young infants, when positioned in prone, have the ability to edge almost imperceptibly from the center of their beds into the corners.

Reciprocal neonatal stepping, requiring considerable external upper body support, is elicited through pedal pressure in the upright position. This behavior is virtually identical to neonatal reciprocal kicking, and the tightly linked leg movements characterizing it in either position may be evident as early as 28 weeks' gestational age. In addition to lifting the feet reciprocally, a positive support reaction is also present in healthy neonates. This is typically elicited by dynamic pressure on the dorsum of the foot followed by pedal loading.

Table 5.1 Emergence of Locomotor Behaviors

Age	Locomotion
10–16 weeks' gestational age	Body rotation relative to umbilical cord as axis
14–15 weeks' gestational age	Crawling/climbing behavior in contact with uterine wall
17–18 weeks' gestational age	Vigorous lower extremity extensor thrusts relative to uterine wall; these continue until birth, but with decreasing vigor as growth and confinement increase
Neonatal period	Neonatal reciprocal stepping when upper body supported; digitigrade in character, with flat foot contact, flexed knees and hips; kinematic pattern identical to kicking pattern in supine Legs display positive support reaction when upper body supported
7–10 weeks	Neonatal stepping disappears unless efforts made to prolong it through practice
Birth–3 months	Quadrupedal extremity efforts, sometimes reciprocal, contribute to change in body position on firm surface when infant positioned in prone; infant positioned in center of bed may be found later snuggled in corner
3–7 months	Pivot prone rotation; infant elevates and rotates upper body in a circular fashion relative to umbilicus as axis
5–7 months	Sequential rolling may be utilized by some infants to locomote
5–7 months	Commando crawling (seal creeping): advancing trunk forward, primarily with arms, present in many infants; typically is next locomotor pattern after pivot-prone rotation
7–9 months	Variety of prewalking locomotor patterns may be observed: scooting on bottom (shuffling or hitching), using one or both arms for support; hands-knees crawling or creeping with abdominal contact; hands-feet crawling or creeping with trunk elevated; lack of uniform agreement across disciplines with respect to definitions of creeping and crawling

Table 5.1 continued

Age	Locomotion
8–11 months	Sidestepping in supported standing (cruising) and transitions while standing among support surfaces in most infants; some infants walk without support; noncrawlers tend to be early walkers unless unusually obese
12 months	Independent walking present in most infants (average age of onset 11.2 months–15 months in various sources); may be characterized by short, uneven steps, wide base of support, absence of knee wave during stance, high guard arm position and many falls; 30% of 1-year-olds can run 15 m (Sutherland, 1988)
18 months	Heel strike replaces flat foot or forefoot at initial contact; reciprocal arm swing present in 50% of children (Rose & Gamble, 1994); 78% can run 15 m (Sutherland, 1988)
2 years	Knee flexion wave consistently present during stance phase; 97% of children can run 15 m; 7% can complete length of a 10 cm × 3 m balance beam with feet placed side by side (Sutherland, 1988)
2 years 6 months	Majority of children can toe-walk; 60% of children can heel-walk; fewer than 5% of children can hop on 1 foot for a distance of 3 m (Sutherland, 1988)
3 years	Most children can heel-walk; 34% can complete length of a 10 cm × 3 m balance beam feet placed side by side (Sutherland, 1988); according to Sutherland, mature gait pattern present, except for increased cadence, decreased step length; mean age of onset of nonsupport phase of running is 33 months (Kucera et al., 1980)
3 years 6 months	Base of support equivalent to or less than pelvic span; 90% of children can heel-walk; 75% of children can complete 10 cm x 3 m balance beam with feet placed side by side
4 years	Reciprocal arm swing should be present in all ambulators; majority of children can hop on 1 foot distance of 3 m; 20% of children can complete 10 cm × 3 m balance beam placing heel of 1 foot directly in front of toes of other (Sutherland, 1988)

Table 5.1 continued

Age	Locomotion
5 years	92% of children can hop on 1 foot distance of 3 m; 80% of children can complete 10 cm × 3 m balance beam with heel of 1 foot directly in front of toes of the other (Sutherland, 1988); ground reaction forces stabilize in the adult pattern (Beck et al., 1981)
6 years	Child should be able to complete 10 cm × 3 m balance beam, placing heel of foot directly in front of toes of other foot (Sutherland, 1988)
7 years	Gait pattern has definitely stabilized in adult mode, but stride length continues to increase with increasing height and leg length

Human neonatal ambulation appears to have no functional purpose, although the same behavior was functionally relevant for the fetus. Unless measures are taken to retain it, for example, walking practice with support, neonatal ambulation disappears around 7–8 weeks of age, to return many months later as a structurally different type of bipedal gait. The absence of a need for neonatal locomotion to continue likely contributes to its disappearance, but continued growth also makes it biomechanically inefficient. Considerable evidence documents that physical parameters determine the type of locomotion selected by humans and animals.

The tightly linked movements of the neonatal hip, knee, and ankle, which permit little or no environmental responsivity, and the abundance of cocontraction characterizing neonatal ambulation also describe the gait pattern seen in children with spastic diplegia. This may represent a form of developmental arrest in a primitive gait pattern.

VARIED ASCENT ROUTES TO INDEPENDENT WALKING

Variations in the developmental ascent pattern are due to an integration of many influences.

1. Culturally related biological differences and caregiving
2. Existence of several possible developmental sequences by which children can attain mature bipedal ambulation
3. Varied physical attributes of growing children which determine preferential selection of certain locomotor behaviors
4. Developmental, neurological, or musculoskeletal disorders

Cultural Differences

Differences present at birth and caregiving practices that lead to selective pressures on motor behavior have been described for several decades (see reviews in Cintas, 1988, 1995). Societies whose caregivers carry their infants in posturally challenging positions and aggressively emphasize the attainment of sitting and standing competence while discouraging crawling may accelerate the appearance of motor milestones by 2–3 months. Societies in which the infant is very protected behaviorally and posturally and the caregiving focus is to optimize comfort and minimize crying contribute to a more relaxed developmental ascent.

Season of Birth

The season in which the child is born may account for differences in the onset of locomotion attributed to other factors. Recent evidence suggests that the lower the temperature during the 6th month following birth, the older infants may be at the onset of locomotion, presumably due to constraint of heavier clothing or absence of floor experience.

Multiple Factors

On the basis of many contributing factors, including biological differences, caregiving, physical parameters, and behavioral attributes such as temperament and motivation, young children select varied locomotor routes to independent walking. Most importantly, at least 12% of children do not crawl or creep before walking; typical children, in fact, precede the development of walking with a variety of locomotor strategies, including bottom scooting. The majority of children do attain quadrupedal locomotion before progressing to bipedal, and these two types of locomotion typically overlap for several months.

Abnormal locomotor development may result from many factors, most of which are related to developmental, neuromotor, or musculoskeletal disorders. These are described in detail in Table 5.2.

GAIT TRANSITIONS WITH MATURATION

Gait Characteristics of Early Independent Walkers

1. Wide base of support
2. Short uneven steps
3. Arms in high guard position
4. Flat foot or forefoot initial contact
5. Increased dorsiflexion during stance
6. Minimal propulsive push-off
7. Significant cocontraction is present in early walkers, which decreases with maturation of the gait pattern.

Table 5.2 Abnormal Locomotor Behaviors

Locomotor Behavior	Contributing Sources	Possible Interventions
Fetal Dyskinesia or Akinesia	Neural tube disorders such as anencephaly and spina bifida	Prenatal monitoring of maternal, embryonic, and fetal status
	Congenital myopathies, neuropathies, or encephalopathies	
	Fetal crowding due to uterine malformation, multiple fetuses, or insufficient amniotic fluid	
	Transient fetal paralysis due to maternal curarization	Avoid paralyzing drugs during gestation
Asymmetrical or Chronic Pivot Prone Rotation	**Normal:** Pivot prone rotation typically precedes crawling/creeping in average infant	
	Abnormal: Infant can rotate to 1 side only or fails to make transition to other forms of locomotion by 9 months; unilateral rotation may be due to one-sided weakness or inappropriate sensory input, for example, visual or vestibular; failure to make transition may be due to inability to weightshift or elevate trunk due to bilateral weakness, hyper or hypotonicity	Precise analysis of barriers or contributing factors guides intervention efforts; essential to address possible sensory contributors to abnormality before instituting vigorous motor intervention

Table 5.2 continued

Locomotor Behavior	Contributing Sources	Possible Interventions
Commando Crawling, also known as Seal Creeping (Single or dual arm-propelled forward locomotion; trunk in contact with support surface; legs typically extended behind)	**Normal:** May be 1st evidence of forward propulsion in average infant; appears just after the onset of pivot prone rotational movements relative to umbilicus as axis **Appropriate:** For child with moderate to severe lower body paralysis, for example, spina bifida **Abnormal:** Does not transition to higher levels of locomotion; persists as only mode of locomotion beyond 9 months of age	Abnormal if due to low tone and inability to elevate trunk over flexed knees: use standing and extension activities to increase general body tone and stability, avoid flexion activities which reduce them Abnormal if due to high lower extremity tone and inability to flex knees under trunk: Utilize rotational transitions such as Sitting to Quadruped to Kneeling to bring tone down, and to promote trunk rotation and extremity dissociation
Bunny Hopping (quadrupedal nonreciprocal locomotion using fully extended bilateral, simultaneous arm support, followed by pulling the flexed knees and hips under the body)	**Normal:** Average child may do this from time to time; child may use this briefly and then make transition to early walking without refining crawling/creeping **Abnormal:** Does not make transition to reciprocal, quadrupedal locomotion or to walking; persists as only method of locomotion beyond 18 months of age with no child-initiated efforts to achieve standing with support	Intervention for abnormality dependent on analysis and identification of factors contributing to absence of reciprocal motion If due to limited hip range of motion, W-sitting only type of sitting and inability to dissociate legs due to high lower extremity muscle tone and dyscoordination: utilize rotational transitions to bring tone down and increase upper and lower extremity dissociation

Table 5.2 continued

Locomotor Behavior	Contributing Sources	Possible Interventions
		If due to poor stability in quadruped: identify source of instability, for example, weakness, insufficient tone, or insufficient balance, and treat accordingly; also provide movement transitions incorporating dissociated extremities and and asymmetrical positions
Bottom Scooting, also known as Bottom Shuffling or Hitching (in sitting, propulsion with flexed legs in front, often using one or both arms for support while moving body forward; rarely, child will do this while positioned in supine)	Sitting version may be chosen by typical children prior to walking; not necessarily abnormal; supine bottom scooting rarely, if ever, observed in average children as frequent or sole mode of locomotion; each is abnormal if persists as only form of locomotion beyond period when child would be expected to achieve standing with support	
Out-toeing during Stance Phase (walking with exaggerated leg external rotation)	**Normal:** During early standing and walking, especially when associated with sidestepping (cruising) and early toddler gait	

Table 5.2 continued

Locomotor Behavior	Contributing Sources	Possible Interventions
Out-toeing during Stance Phase (cont)	**Abnormal:** Associated with muscle weakness and connective tissue laxity leading to instability in standing May be a compensation to promote knee extension stability or ankle alignment stability during stance phase; contributing conditions include spina bifida, poliomyelitis, lower motorneuron and intrinsic muscle disorders Symptomatic of slipped capital femoral epiphysis (SCFE), especially when unilateral Associated with femoral retroversion, calcaneal malalignment	Analysis of source of problem critical to choice of intervention; bracing to improve ankle stability or derotation cables mounted on pelvic band to improve knee alignment may be considered Hip external rotation may contribute to hip stability in children with flaccid paralysis; bias toward external rotation may be beneficial in some cases if ankles well aligned Surgical interventions may be appropriate for SCFE or extreme femoral retroversion
In-toeing during Stance Phase (walking with exaggerated leg internal rotation)	**Normal:** Peak period of anteversion in children occurs between 1–3 years of age; some children may show transient in-toeing associated with this during this period; spontaneous correction can occur even beyond 8 years of age (Sutherland, 1984) Genetically transmitted in families; high incidence in fast runners	Analysis of contributing factors includes differentiation between soft tissue contributors and structural contributors; if ankle instability or severe malalignment exists in standing, must be addressed first through exercise, bracing, or surgery before knee or hip joints can be accurately evaluated; however, hip and/or knee malalignment may be manifested at the ankle

Table 5.2 continued

Locomotor Behavior	Contributing Sources	Possible Interventions
In-toeing during Stance Phase (cont)	**Abnormal:** Many sources of abnormality contribute to in-toeing individually or in combination. They include: muscle weakness or tonal imbalance leading to hip internal rotation bias, hip subluxation or dislocation, increased femoral anteversion; medial knee rotation due to weakness or ligamentous laxity, medial tibial torsion, forefoot varus, midfoot pronation or supination and hindfoot elevation, and calcaneal eversion or inversion	Combination of hip internal rotation bias, femoral anteversion, medial tibial rotation or torsion, medial midfoot collapse, and calcaneal eversion or inversion often associated with spastic cerebral palsy. May be considerably minimized with infant treatment to balance movement patterns and tone prior to standing; once standing introduced, emphasis on activating full hip extension in standing, and linking hip extension with hip abduction, hip external rotation, knee extension, and ankle dorsiflexion while standing and walking
Genu Varus Gait (bow legged gait)	**Normal:** Often, but not consistently, observed in young toddlers up to 2 years of age; spontaneous correction is typical	
	Abnormal: Normal conversion from tibial varus to valgus fails to occur; creates abnormal compression forces on medial tibia (Blount Disease)	Bracing or early surgical osteotomy necessary to intervene in progression of Blount disease

Table 5.2 continued

Locomotor Behavior	Contributing Sources	Possible Interventions
Genu Valgus Gait (knock kneed gait)	**Normal:** Maximal tibial valgal angle around 3 years of age; progressive reduction occurs up to approximately 6½ years of age	
	Abnormal: Rare but occasionally seen in conjunction with severe rheumatoid arthritis, more commonly in adults	Rheumatoid Arthritis: monitor tendency with growth; intervene early with asymmetrical knee strengthening exercise, joint preservation techniques, and night splints; consider ankle orthoses positioned in supination
Toe Walking	**Normal:** Average children may experiment with toe walking for brief periods, but it is not part of evolution of normal gait	
	Abnormal: Idiopathic toe walkers may have no signs of neurologial disorder, stand statically with their heels down, and elevate only when walking	Idiopathic toe walking typically responds to developmental activities, exercises, casting, or bracing
	Toe walking can be early indication of muscular dystrophy, spinal muscular atrophy, cerebral palsy or, if unilateral, hip dislocation	Comprehensive diagnostic testing important to rule out neurological disesase; dynamic EMG may be useful to distinguish idiopathic toe walkers

Table 5.2 continued

Locomotor Behavior	Contributing Sources	Possible Interventions
Equinus Gait (exaggerated plantar flexion of the foot during swing; forefoot contact during stance)	Typically due to specific equinovarus deformity resulting from congenital clubfoot or severely shortened achilles tendon as a result of chronic muscle imbalance Deformity may be a gait stabilizer during stance; crouch gait may result if ankle and foot alignment corrected	Rarely if ever responds to exercise as primary intervention; serial casting may be effective, but at risk of damaging midfoot medial arch; surgery followed by bracing often utilized for correction
Crouch Gait (excessive hip and knee flexion, ankle dorsiflexion during stance phase)	Commonly attributed to overzealous heel cord lengthening in children with spastic cerebral palsy, but may be due to multiple factors, including: • Inability to achieve extension due to weakness or hypotonia • Inability to achieve extension due to hip and knee flexor spasticity • Biomechanical disadvantage created by achilles tendon lengthening when significant hamstrings spasticity present	Analysis of source critical to choice of intervention; exercise may be effective to address weakness, hypotonia, or hypertonia; posterior entry bracing with anterior ankle support may improve alignment and function
Calcaneal Gait (flat-footed gait without push-off)	Typically due to flaccid paralysis or absence of sensation; may occur in conjunction with crouch gait	Exercise rarely sufficient to increase strength; stretching of soft tissue structures may lead to further decompensation; consider bracing to protect ankle with stop to limit dorsiflexion and facilitate push-off

Table 5.2 continued

Locomotor Behavior	Contributing Sources	Possible Interventions
Trendelenberg Gait (exaggerated lateral pelvic elevation associated with pelvic drop on opposite side; defined here as intrinsic pelvic elevation or trunk lateral shift to elevate pelvis)	Typically due to leg length discrepancy or scoliosis in children May be associated with hip abductor weakness leading to gluteus medius lurch: • Following late diagnosis of congenital hip dislocation • Bilateral in children with intrinsic muscle disease who may need exaggerated trunk lateral shifts in order to advance leg in swing phase	Analyze and remediate source; discriminate structural cause such as leg length discrepancy versus muscle weakness
	Occasionally due to poor prosthetic fit or performance; child shifts trunk laterally to clear prosthesis Occasionally due to fused joint or antalgic gait	Discriminate between prosthetic structural problem or fit and child's inability to perform well with prosthesis due to weakness or dyscoordination
	May be necessary to advance bilateral long leg braces	Investigate lighter weight bracing system, parapodium, or reciprocal cable orthosis

Gait Transitions

1. Wide base of support decreases to within the confines of pelvic span (reported to occur at 17½ weeks to 3½ years after onset of independent walking).
2. Increased gait velocity is due to increased cadence **during the transition** from supported to independent walking.
3. Increased gait velocity is due to increased stride length **after onset** of independent walking; cadence decreases with age
   a. Tables correlating stride length with age are available in many sources
   b. Several authors have suggested that leg length, in association with height, more accurately predicts stride length
   c. Beck and colleagues (1981) reported that average stride length was equivalent to 76% of a child's height, irrespective of age, at a standard walking speed
   d. Sutherland (1988) counters that the correlation between leg length and age is 0.95 between 1 and 7 years of age.
4. Transition from toddler's high guard arm position to reciprocal arm swing occurs 4–5 months after the onset of independent walking (range of 6–43 weeks)
   a. Not evident before 1 year of age
   b. Present in 50% of children by 18 months of age
   c. Should be present in all children by 4 years of age.
5. Flat foot initial contact and excessive hip flexion in toddlers transitions to appearance of heel strike at an average of 22 ½ weeks after the onset of independent walking.
   a. Initial contact should consistently be heel strike in the average child by 18 months of age
   b. Flat foot contact and excessive hip flexion beyond 23 months is abnormal
6. Excessive cocontraction linking the early toddler's lower extremity joints is gradually replaced by more mature phasic patterns
   a. Plantar flexion of the ankle and simultaneous flexion of the knee, which permit the knee flexion wave during stance, appear about 15 weeks after the onset of independent walking; should be present by 2 years of age
   b. Dorsiflexion of the ankle now occurs in conjunction with knee extension at the end of swing phase, facilitating heel strike.

In general, the transition from toddler to more mature gait patterns begins at the hip and moves distally to the ankle. A lack of uniformity exists in the literature as to when the transition process is completed; various sources indicate a range from 3–7 years of age.

DEVELOPMENTAL CHANGES IN POSTURAL CONTROL OR BALANCE

Perspectives of locomotor development from the standpoint of increasing growth, maturation, or accumulated experience are, by necessity, hierarchical. In contrast, the distributed control, or dynamic systems model, views the developing child as utilizing perception to identify salient aspects of the environment, and acting on them. This is supported by a nervous system that can respond at multiple levels of demand.

1. Vision is critical to the development of the postural control necessary for locomotion in infants.
   a. Infants as young as 2 months of age respond with appropriate head movement to movement of the walls and ceiling of a room
   b. This sensitivity declines with the onset of crawling at about 6 months of age
   c. Same sensitivity is again evident when standing is acquired, but it decreases with time and the acquisition of walking experience
   d. Vision appears to be the dominant perceptual means of modulating posture at each major transition
      - Sitting to crawling
      - Crawling to standing
      - Standing to walking.
2. Children's postural responses assessed while standing on a moving platform vary considerably with age and experience in standing, as described by Woolacott et al. in 1989.
   a. From 8–14 months of age
      - No response in the youngest nonstanders
      - Followed by inconsistent responses in the lower leg with increasing age
      - Consistent responses in the lower leg by 14 months of age
   b. From 15 months–3 years of age
      - Distal muscles are consistently activated before proximal muscles, the pattern seen in adults
      - Responses are larger in amplitude and longer in latency and duration than those of adults.
   c. Children's postural responses from 4–6 years of age appear to regress
      - Leg response synergies are more variable and of longer latency than younger or older children
      - Neck flexor muscle responses occur less frequently than in younger children and adults and, when present, are highly variable
      - Trunk extensor muscles also display longer latency than those seen in younger children.

Wollacott and colleagues (1989) have suggested that this apparent regression may represent a period during which children are integrating visual, vestibular, and somatosensory inputs influencing posture and balance. In this way, the dominance of vision may gradually decrease, fostering the transition to reliance on sensory systems other than vision, which is characteristic of adults. In fact, children from 7–10 years of age demonstrate adaptive postural responses similar to those of adults.

Although young children rely heavily on visual information for postural adjustments during locomotor development, postural responses are present in all age groups when visual cues are eliminated. In some instances, response latencies to perturbation decrease in the absence of vision, suggesting that removal of visual information may increase the sensitivity to the remaining proprioceptive and vestibular cues. While vision appears to become less dominant with increasing age, it nonetheless occupies an increasingly important role as the means of discriminating among conflicting environmental cues.

COMPONENTS OF MATURE AMBULATION

Descriptive terms relating to gait are not uniformly defined in the literature. These appear to be the definitions most generally applied:

1. **Cadence:** number of steps per minute; average values are 175 at 1 year of age, 153 at 3 years of age, 143 at 7 years of age, and 114 in adults.
2. **Gait cycle or walking cycle:** completed cycle of both feet, typically from right foot strike to right foot strike
3. **Initial contact:** foot strike, heel strike, or heel contact
4. **Pelvic rotation:** rotation of pelvis which accompanies relative forward (swing) and backward (stance) movement of each leg
5. **Pelvic tilt:** lateral elevation or depression of pelvis in the frontal plane; also known as pelvic list
6. **Stance phase:** equivalent to 60–62% of total gait cycle; further subdivided into:
   - **Initial or early double support (loading period):** from foot strike (initial contact) to toe-off of opposite foot
   - **Single limb stance:** opposite leg in swing phase
   - **Second or late double support (pre-swing period):** from heel strike of opposite foot to toe-off of target foot
7. **Step length:** distance measured from heel of 1 foot to heel of other foot when both feet on the ground at the same time
8. **Stride length:** sum of left and right step lengths
9. **Stride time:** duration of complete gait cycle
10. **Swing phase:** equivalent to 38–40% of gait cycle; begins with toe-off (lift off) and ends with foot strike or initial contact of next cycle; can be further subdivided into:
    - **Acceleration phase**
    - **Midswing**
    - **Deceleration phase**
11. **Toe in or toe out angle:** angle in degrees between the direction of progression and a reference line on sole of foot, commonly its midline, usually measured on a contact footprint
12. **Walking velocity:** average speed in single direction, in cm/sec or m/min; average values: 64 cm/sec at 1 year of age, 86 cm/sec at 3 years of age, 114 cm/sec at 7 years of age, and 122 cm/sec for adults; actual velocity more dependent on height and leg length than age.

GAIT ASSESSMENT

Gait assessment is critical for the evaluation of children's baseline function and change in performance. Means of assessment have evolved from strictly visual observation to highly technical recording and evaluative methods. These are described in Table 5.3.

Table 5.3 Motion, Primarily Gait, Assessment Methods

Type	Description	Advantages and Limitations
Visual Inspection (observational gait analysis)	Visual evaluation of gait parameters; should include anterior, lateral, and posterior placement of observer relative to moving child	Naturalistic, minimal intrusion on child's spontaneous behavior; can be immediately applied and ongoing; can be used to guide treatment decisions and intervention during treatment session Recording of observations by progress note or by communication to child, family, or colleagues; locomotor behavior not documented in a reproducible way for comparison with subsequent evaluations More consistent with single than multiple observers; events lasting < $\frac{1}{16}$ sec duration or at multiple joints cannot be accurately captured by human eye
Videotaping or Cinematography	Dynamic recording of locomotion using videotaping or motion picture camera	Provides documentation of visual gait evaluation, which, if carried out in a reproducible manner, can be used for comparison; in conjunction with other gait evaluation techniques, can be valuable method of recording in a standardized fashion

Table 5.3 continued

Type	Description	Advantages and Limitations
Videotaping or Cinematography (cont)		If camera placement not carefully considered in relation to child's position, may be of little value, especially if each recording session not performed in standard fashion in terms of sequence; may be useful to record temporal aspects of gait, but degree of error in recording and playback systems difficult to assess and control for unless timer is incorporated into frames
Digitizing	Method of determining joint angles; can be applied to videotaped data to provide kinematic information on static joint position and changing joint angles; can also be coordinated with other types of gait evaluation done in laboratory; if skin markers used with good background contrast, automatic tracking of marker positions and digitizing possible while taping with some systems	Can increase value of videotaped data significantly if joint angle measurements are desired; computer software programs available for this purpose following videotaping, although it can be done manually Value and accuracy of digitizing depends on value of videotaped data; camera placement in relation to movement is critical; may require up to 3–4 cameras

Table 5.3 continued

Type	Description	Advantages and Limitations
Foot print Recording	Many inexpensive approaches, including stepping in water and walking across firm surface, stepping in powder and walking on continuous paper from large roll; child can step in ink or paint before walking on paper; paper which is treated to respond to foot placement with a permanent visual display can be purchased (Examples: Shutrak or Fuji Prescale)	In conjunction with videotaping, can provide comprehensive means of objective gait assessment in treatment setting; can measure step and stride length, base of support, and toe out or toe in angle; using stopwatch, can also measure temporal parameters such as velocity and cadence
Mirrored Plexiglass Standing Frame or Walking Surface	Foot contact patterns can be photographed in standing, and occasionally during walking	Relatively inexpensive means of recording foot pressure by photography; generally limited to static standing Limited data yield in proportion to equipment expense, although may be useful for guidance in orthotic fabrication and adjustment
Pedobarograph	Means of measuring pressure beneath foot during gait using an elastic mat on top of an edge-lit glass plate; pressure during walking compresses mat onto glass differentially, decreasing reflectivity in proportion to increased pressure; monochrome image under glass processed into color image corresponding to different levels of pressure	Generally available in gait laboratory; data much more elaborate and precise than from other foot contact pressure methods, but at considerably greater expense; graphic aspects of data display useful for formal presentation or publication

Table 5.3 continued

Type	Description	Advantages and Limitations
Force Platform or Force Plate Recording	Measures ground reaction forces as ambulator walks over it, providing kinetic data; consists of rigid surface with underlying transducers that measure surface displacement in 3 axes; ideally mounted flush with walkway; data collected by microcomputer; force plate data can also be utilized to evaluate energy changes occurring as center of mass rises and falls	Used mainly when ground reaction force data combined with kinematic information; sources of error include failure to shield system from outside influences and inability of platform to respond accurately when full foot not on platform
Instrumented Walkway	Instrumentation is within walkway, not on walker; used to measure timing and placement of foot contact; if used with photoelectric beams, can also measure gait velocity; switch contacts are within walkway itself; or, electrical contacts on walker's shoes (requiring cable attachment) close circuit with conductive substance on walkway	Data collection done by microcomputer, but system can be expensive and unreliable because of switch contact malfunction; in-shoe placement of switches may provide similar data at considerably less cost
Electrogoniometry	Direct measurement devices applied to child; 2 types of electrogoniometers most often employed are potentiometers and flexible strain gauges; give kinematic data relating joint angles and time, or angular relationships of more than 1 joint	Direct measurement of joint rotation, multiple goniometers can be mounted in several planes in an attempt to provide 3-D recording Multiple error sources include invasive nature of recording on child's behavior

Table 5.3 continued

Type	Description	Advantages and Limitations
	Most commonly used for knee, and less often for hip and ankle; trailing wires or cables transmit data to microcomputer	and difficulty of aligning goniometer with true joint axis in a dynamic situation; even multiple goniometers may not capture degrees of freedom in a joint; digitizing with videotaping or optical kinematic recording may be preferable for most children
Electromyography	Direct measurement of muscle activation patterns, generally used in conjunction with simultaneous recording of other gait parameters; superficial electrodes most commonly used; data collected and integrated by means of microcomputer requiring trailing cable attached to moving child or use of telemetry unit; fine wire or needle electrodes provide more specificity for individual muscle recording, but typically not used for gait analysis, especially in children	Abundant amount of normative EMG data for all age groups provides valuable means for comparison; little value if isolated from time points in gait cycle because provides information about electrical activity, not mechanical activation; crosstalk among adjacent muscles makes inferences about group activity relatively accurate, but not for individual muscles Movement potential source of error as well as external sources of artifact
Kinematic Systems	Used to record position of body segments, angles of joints, and corresponding velocities and accelerations; several options available: photographic systems or videographic systems with digitizing capability, television/computer systems utilizing re-	Provide abundant opportunities for data collection on multiple joint movements under laboratory-controlled conditions; especially useful for investigative purposes and baseline gait analysis prior to orthopedic surgery; data collection and integration

Table 5.3 continued

Type	Description	Advantages and Limitations
	flective markers providing reconstruction of data in 3-D on television screen, opticoelectric systems using light-emitting diodes as joint markers which are coded by an opticoelectric camera, and opticoelectronic scanners using passive reflective markers which are color-coded to indicate marker positions	carried out by microcomputer but still quite labor intensive; trained personnel essential, full-time engineer often necessary for hardware management; expensive to set up and maintain; intimidating environment for child, may influence performance
Combined Kinematic and Kinetic Motion Analysis Systems	Provide ability to combine force plate (kinetic) data with kinematic information, allowing limb segment to be evaluated as total mechanical system	Crème de la crème of motion analysis systems; very expensive; can be intimidating for all except the very courageous; multiple sources of breakdown and error; an engineer within shouting distance is essential
Assessment of Energy Costs of Locomotion	Several methods available: measurement of oxygen consumption and/or carbon dioxide production using a gas measurement and collection system; estimation of energy cost using kinematic data by estimating mass of body parts x distance traveled x acceleration; monitoring heart rate as a function of speed to determine physiological cost index; and, using kinetic data (ground reaction forces) as well as kinematic data to estimate energy cost with inverse dynamics calculations (Winter, 1979)	

6 / Administrative Issues

Toby M. Long

In an era of increased emphasis on accountability for continuing services, effective documentation is a significant concern for providers. Additionally, physical therapy for infants and children is provided in a variety of environments such as hospitals, public and private schools, rehabilitation centers, and in the home. Within these environments, there are often various levels of care which are based on seriousness of illness, purpose of agency providing service, needs of the family, and the accessibility of service provision. The purpose of this chapter is to review the philosophical, legislative, and regulatory issues influencing service delivery, to describe various service delivery environments available, and to present information on the documentation systems often used when providing physical therapy to children with disabilities.

PHILOSOPHICAL UNDERPINNINGS

Although the provision of physical therapy to children varies across jurisdictions and environments, most pediatric physical therapy is grounded on five major premises which guide the design of interventions and service delivery.

First Three Years

The first three years of life are critical in the development of a child. The interaction between the child and the environment during this time lays the foundation for future communication and cognition, social relationships, and adaptive performance.

Children As Active Learners

Children's needs and interests must be taken into account in designing treatment and service delivery. Participation by the child and his or her family is necessary within treatment sessions as well as for decision-making regarding service delivery.

Intervention Evolves

Intervention is most successful when begun as soon as possible and when the child and family are available to participate actively. Intervention will evolve over time to meet the changing needs of the child and family.

External Factors

External factors, even if temporary, can influence the development of a child. These factors, which include the child's family, culture, environment, and the social system, must be accounted for when designing an intervention program.

The Family

The family is the constant in the child's life. Treatment must involve the family at all levels of decision-making, and physical therapists must develop a collaborative relationship with the family.

LEGISLATIVE DIRECTION

Education

1. Individuals with Disabilities Education Act (IDEA) (1993) (PL 102–119). Describes the requirements of educational and early intervention services to children with disabilities. IDEA encompasses the original Education of the Handicapped Act (PL 94–142) and its amendments (PL 99–457). Three categories of service requirements are described in the law and subsequent regulations. These categories are based on the age of the child. Part B of the act describes the services to be provided to children aged 6–21 years (school age). This is the original PL 94–142 passed by Congress in 1975. It requires that all states provide a free and appropriate public education (FAPE) for children with disabilities. The education plan is an individualized education plan (IEP). Physical therapy is considered a related service and thus is only provided to assist with the accomplishment of a child's educational goals. Part B also describes the services that are provided to children aged 3–5 years (preschoolers). Part H describes the services to children from birth–2 years of age (infants and toddlers). Significant features of the act pertaining to the three age groups are compared in Table 6.1.
2. Technology-Related Assistance for Individuals with Disabilities Act ("The Tech Act") (PL 100–407). Recognizes the need for assistive technology (wheelchairs, communication systems) for children with disabilities and authorizes funding for states to create statewide systems of technological assistance.
3. The Carl D. Perkins Vocational and Applied Technology Education Act (1990). Requires individuals with disabilities to be provided with vocational education in the least restrictive environment (LRE). When appropriate, vocational education is part of IEP.

Rehabilitation/Civil Rights

1. Americans with Disabilities Act (ADA) (1990) (PL 101–336). Assures that people with disabilities are afforded equal access and reasonable accommodation in employment and services provided by both private and public sectors.
   a. Prohibits the imposition on applications of eligibility criteria that screen out or tend to screen out individuals with disabilities
   b. Prohibits the exclusion and segregation of individuals with disabilities and the denial of opportunities enjoyed by others
   c. Separate, special, or different programs that are designed to provide benefit to persons with disabilities cannot be used to restrict the participation of persons with disabilities in general integrated activities.

Table 6.1. Comparison of Part B and Part H of IDEA

Issue	Part B		Part H
	School Age	Preschool	Infant/Toddler
Eligible Children	6–21 year-olds: 1) Having mental retardation, hearing impairment, visual impairment, serious emotional disturbance, orthopedic impairments, autism, traumatic brain injury, other health impairments, specific learning disabilities 2) Who need special education and related service	3–5 year–olds: 1) Having mental retardation, hearing impairment, visual impairment, serious emotional disturbance, orthopedic impairments, autism, traumatic brain injury, other health impairments, specific learning disabilities 2) At state's discretion children showing developmental delays in the following areas: • Physical • Cognitive • Communication • Social or emotional • Adaptive 3) Who need special education and related services	Birth–2 year–olds: 1) Showing developmental delays (as defined by state) in the following areas: • Cognitive • Physical • Communication • Social or emotional • Adaptive 2) Having a diagnosed physical or mental condition which has a high probability of resulting in developmental delay 3) "At-risk" for developmental delay at state's discretion 4) Who are in need of early intervention
Services	Special education and related services documented on Individualized Education Program (IEP) include but are not limited to:		Early intervention services documented on Individualized Family Service Plans (IFSP) include but are not limited to:

Table 6.1. continued

Issue	Part B: School Age / Preschool	Part H: Infant/Toddler
	• Audiology • Counseling services (services by qualified social workers or other[s]) • Medical services (for diagnostic purposes) • Occupational therapy • Parent counseling and training • Physical therapy* • Psychological services • Recreation • School health services (provided by a school nurse or other qualified person) • Speech pathology • Transportation * Physical therapy is considered a related service, and thus is only provided to assist in meeting the educational plan	• Audiology • Service coordination • Family training, and counseling • Health services • Medical services (for diagnostic purposes) • Nursing services • Nutrition services • Occupational therapy • Physical therapy* • Psychological services • Social work services • Special instruction • Speech-language pathology • Early identification, screening, and assessment • Vision services • Assistive technology devices • Transportation * Physical therapy is considered an early intervention service, and thus can be provided irrespective of the educational goals for the child

Table 6.1. continued

Issue	Part B: School Age	Part B: Preschool	Part H: Infant/Toddler
Individualized Plans	Individualized Education Program (IEP): • Child's present levels of educational performance • Annual goals, including short-term instructional objectives • Specific special education and related services to be provided to the child, and the extent to which the child will be able to participate in regular education programs • Dates for initiation of services and the anticipated duration of the services • Appropriate, objective criteria and evaluation procedures and schedules for determining, on at least an annual basis, whether the short-term instructional objectives are being achieved • Transition services		Individualized Family Service Plan (IFSP): • Child's present levels of development • A family-directed assessment of the resources, priorities, and concerns of the family • Major outcomes child and family are expected to achieve, and the criteria, procedures, and timelines used to determine: 1) Degree to which progress toward achieving the outcome is being made; and 2) Whether modifications or revisions of the outcomes or services are necessary
	• At age 16 every student will have an explicitly written plan for transition into employment or postsecondary education	• At local or state discretion, and with the concurrence of the family, 3–5 year—olds may have an IFSP vs. IEP, so long as IEP requirements are met	

Table 6.1. continued

	Part B		Part H
Issue	School Age	Preschool	Infant/Toddler
			• Statement of the specific early intervention services necessary to meet the unique needs of the child and family to achieve the outcomes identified, including: 1) Frequency, intensity, location, and method of delivering services 2) Payment arrangements, if any 3) Other services not required by this act but needed by the child, and steps to secure these services from other sources • Projected dates for initiation of services and the anticipated duration of those services • Name of the service coordinator who is qualified to carry out the responsibilities of the position under Part H

Table 6.1. continued

Issue	Part B: School Age	Part B: Preschool	Part H: Infant/Toddler
			• Steps to be taken to support the transition of the child at age 3 • Statement of the natural environments in which early intervention services shall be provided • Requires informed, written consent from parents before services in !FSP are provided. If parents do not provide consent for all services, services for which consent is given must be provided.
Integration	Least Restricted Environment: "to the maximum extent appropriate, children with disabilities, . . . are educated with children who are not disabled, and that special classes, separate schooling, or other removal of children with disabilities from the regular educational environment occurs only when the nature or severity of the disability is such that education in regular classes with the use of supplementary aids and services cannot be achieved satisfactorily"		"to the maximum extent appropriate, [services] are provided in natural environments, including the home and community settings . . . in which children without disabilities participate"
Lead Agency	State education agency		Governor-designated lead agency

Table 6.1. continued

Issue	Part B: School Age	Part B: Preschool	Part H: Infant/Toddler

Advisory Panels	State Special Education Advisory Panel:
	• Appointed by Governor
	• Members include:
	  • Consumers
	  • Parents
	  • Teachers
	  • Special education administrators
	  • State and local officials
			Interagency Coordinating Council:
			• Appointed by Governor
			• At least 15 members but no more than 25 (unless approved)
			• Members include:
			  • 20% parents
			  • 20% providers
			  • 1 legislator
			  • 1 personnel trainer
			  • 1 state education agency
			  • Representative of the 3–5 program
			  • 1 state insurance representative
			  • Chair may be appointed by Governor from the members, or the Governor shall have the members designate; no lead agency representative may serve as chair
			• May have birth–5 years focus
			• Shall advise on transition
			• Establishes a Federal Interagency Coordinating Council

Table 6.1. continued

	Part B		Part H
Issue	School Age	Preschool	Infant/Toddler
Participation of Other Agencies	Must meet state standards and be under general supervision of State education agency		Must meet state standards and be under general supervision of lead agency
Implementation Timeline	All eligible children must be receiving services by FY 1991 (school year 1991–1992) or sanctions are applied		• All eligible children must be receiving services no later than beginning of state's 5th year of participation in program if the state continues to participate • Provides for "differential funding," which authorizes a maximum of 2 one–year extensions for states that are unable to meet their fifth–year requirements within 5 years of participation if the Governor requests an extension and the Secretary grants it; funding is at a reduced level for those states awarded extensions

Table 6.1. continued

Issue	Part B: School Age	Part B: Preschool	Part H: Infant/Toddler
Application for Funds	State education agency applies every 3 years		Lead agency applies every year and every 3 years after full implementation
Basis for Allocation of Dollars to State	Preschool children generate funding from both the Part B State Grant Program and the Part B—Section 619 (Preschool) Program Each state receives funds in proportion to the number of 3–21 year-olds served on December 1 of the previous year; no state shall receive less than $40,000 for administration. Preschool grants authorized up to $1500 per child		Each state receives funds in proportion to its general population of birth–2 year-olds, not less than $500,000
State Use of Funds	At least 75% of funds must flow to local education agencies on a prorated basis; up to 20% of funds may be used at state's discretion; up to 5% of funds may be used for administrative purposes; shall not supplant; use for "excess cost"		To plan, develop, and implement statewide system of services; funds cannot be used for services that are provided or paid for through other sources; Part H funds are payor of last resort and are to be distributed equitably across geographic areas
	Allows for flexible use of both Part B and Part H funds during the year the child turns 3 years of age; allows for the use of both Part B and Part H funds for the planning of a B-5 seamless system of services.		

Table 6.1. continued

	Part B		Part H
Issue	School Age	Preschool	Infant/Toddler
Cost to Parents	No cost to parents (FAPE)		State must establish a sliding fee scale if state law permits; however, families may not be denied services because of inability to pay; certain services must be provided at no cost: child find, evaluation and assessment, service coordination, development and review of IFSP, and procedural safeguards; if a state provides "a free, appropriate public education" (FAPE) from birth, all services are at no charge

2. Rehabilitation Act Amendment of 1992 (PL 102–569). Revises and extends the programs of the Rehabilitation Act of 1973 (including Section 504). Provisions ensure that the individual served is involved in the development of the Individual Written Rehabilitation Plan (IWRP). Clarifies that vocational rehabilitation services include personal assistance, transition, and supported employment.

Medicaid

1. Catastrophic Coverage Act (1988) (PL 100–360). Allows states to obtain limited funds for services described in a child's IEP or IFSP.
2. Medicaid Amendments (1989) (PL 101–239). Under the Omnibus Budget Reconciliation Act (OBRA), expands Early and Periodic Screening, Diagnosis, and Treatment (EPSDT) and allows Medicaid funds for "medically necessary" treatment.

TEAM COMPOSITION AND DYNAMICS

Because the development of a child crosses disciplinary boundaries, the use of a team of professionals is advocated to meet the diverse needs of the child. A team consists of two or more individuals who provide intervention to an individual and his or her family. Table 6.2 compares the three common types of team composition (multidisciplinary, interdisciplinary, and transdisciplinary).

Transdisciplinary teams require team members to "role release," to share responsibilities and roles across disciplines. Discipline-specific objectives incorporated into an overall intervention plan necessitate the teaching of discipline-specific skills to another. The responsibility of monitoring the plan, updating the strategies, and monitoring the performance of the skills by the team is done by the professional in accordance with the laws and ethics governing their practice. Table 6.3 compares the roles of the therapist on a transdisciplinary team versus an interdisciplinary team.

SERVICE DELIVERY

Driving Forces of Service Delivery

1. System-centered: the strengths and needs of the system drive the delivery of services.
2. Child-centered: the strengths and needs of the child drive the delivery of services.
3. Family-centered: The strengths and needs of the family drive the delivery of services.

Service Delivery Environments

A child with a disability or who is at risk for developing a disability due to environmental or biological complications often receives physical therapy throughout many years and within many environments. Although treatment is individualized to meet the unique needs of each child and his or her family, the purpose of treatment and the design of a treatment plan are often dependent on the service delivery environment. The following will outline the distinct features of pediatric physical therapy within specific environments.

1. Hospital
   a. Neonatal intensive care unit (NICU). To provide developmental support to an infant when medically stable. Positioning programs, environmental adaptations, and incorporation of neuromotor activities into daily caregiving routines are the primary treatment strategies. Strong emphasis of physical therapist working collaboratively with nurses and medical staff to minimize handling of the infant.
   b. Pediatric acute care. Purpose is to decrease pain and discomfort, to diminish effects on function from an acute illness or injury, and to prepare child for discharge. The traditional unidisciplinary medical model of service delivery is common, although small multidisciplinary team models may be utilized. Discipline-specific treatment plans.
   c. Rehabilitation center. Comprehensive and intensive treatment service utilizing a multidisciplinary team approach. Emphasis on improving functional skills through exercise, activity, and adaptive equipment.
   d. Outpatient. Usually short-term services for children recovering from an acute illness or injury. For children with long-term disabilities, treatment as a hospital outpatient is often a transitional service prior to the arrangement of community-based outpatient, early intervention, educationally based, or rehabilitation services to meet the needs of child and family.
2. Early Intervention (EI)

EI services are designed for children from birth to three years and may encompass services provided to children in hospitals, especially NICU, or transitional care units. EI services are described by IDEA under Part H (see Table 6.1). As EI services are guided by a family-centered philosophy, services can be provided in a variety of settings such as child care centers, the home, hospital, or a specific EI program. EI describes a system of care promoting inclusion rather than a care environment. It requires collaboration among services providers and interagency cooperation to prevent duplication of services and promote consistency among service providers. Physical therapy is considered a primary service provider. The purpose of therapy within this context is to enhance the child's functional skills and is outcome-based.

Depending on the age of the child and degree of functional impairment, physical therapy may be provided as a single service or within an interdisciplinary or transdisciplinary team model. Team members can include parents and child care providers in addition to the traditional services providers (educators, occupational therapists, physicians, and speech language pathologists).

Therapeutic plans are incorporated into an Individualized Family Service Plan (IFSP) (Fig. 6.1). Specific treatment goals and objectives are derived from outcomes established by the team utilizing a top-down assessment approach rather than a reductionist, deficit model, or bottom-up assessment approach (see Chapter 2).

Table 6.2. Service Provision Teams

	Multidisciplinary	Interdisciplinary	Trandisciplinary
Assessment	Separate assessments by team members	Separate assessments by team members	Team members and family conduct a comprehensive developmental assessment together
Parent Participation	Parents meet with individual team members	Parents meet with team or team representative	Parents are full, active, and participating members of the team
Service Plan Development	Team members develop separate plans for their disciplines	Team members share their separate plans with one another	Team members and the parents develop a service plan based upon family priorities, needs, and resources
Service Plan Responsibility	Team members are responsible for implementing their sections of the plan	Team members are responsible for sharing information with one another as well as for implementing their section of the plan	Team members are responsible and accountable for how the primary service provider implements the plan
Service Plan Implementation	Team members implement the part of the service plan related to their disciplines	Team members implement their section of the plan and incorporate other sections where possible	A primary service provider is assigned to implement the plan with the family

Table 6.2. continued

	Multidisciplinary	Interdisciplinary	Trandisciplinary
Lines of Communication	Informal lines	Periodic case—specific team meetings	Regular team meetings where continuous transfer of information, knowledge, and skills are shared among team members
Guiding Philosophy	Team members recognize the importance of contributions from other disciplines	Team members are willing and able to develop, share, and be responsible for providing services that are a part of the total service plan	Team members make a commitment to teach, learn, and work together across discipline boundaries to implement unified service plan
Staff Development	Independent and within their disciplines	Independent within as well as outside of their disciplines	An integral component of team meetings is for learning across disciplines and team building

Table 6.3. Comparison of Therapist's Roles in Interdisciplinary and Transdisciplinary Team Models

Case: Jenny, 18-month-old child, with a diagnosis of right hemiplegia, is beginning to ambulate. She prefers to use her left arm because movement in her right arm is difficult. She does not cross midline, transfer objects, or reach above her head with her right arm. Her range of motion is limited in her shoulder, making dressing difficult.

Interdisciplinary Team Model	Transdisciplinary Team Model
Developmental goal: Jenny will reach out and grab a doll from the toy shelf in 7 out of 10 trials with her right arm.	Outcome: Jenny will be able to push both arms through her jacket or into an over-the-head shirt during dressing in all settings.
Physical therapy goal: Jenny will increase the range of motion of right shoulder flexion by 10°.	
Activities	Activities
A. Jenny will be requested and encouraged to reach up and grab her doll from the shelf with her right arm (setting: infant program).	A. During circle time, one teacher-directed activity will be chosen that requires the children to reach above their heads to carry an object or clap, etc. During the activity, the primary service provider will passively move Jenny's arm through full range of motion, incorporating gentle shoulder joint mobility. Therapist will instruct primary service provider in proper range-of-motion and mobilization techniques. (Therapist will monitor these activities weekly.)
B. Jenny will receive passive range-of-motion exercises with mobilization to her right shoulder (setting: physical therapy room twice weekly for ½ hour sessions).	B. Similar routines will be carried out prior to and as needed throughout tabletop activities, prior to feeding, and when it is time to put on and remove clothing (setting: home and center).
C. Parents will be taught range-of-motion exercises to be done each evening prior to bed (setting: home).	

Table 6.3. continued

	C. Jenny will be positioned in prone with arms over a wedge or roll, encouraging full shoulder-forward flexion during a fine motor or art activity. Prior to the activity, the primary service provider will provide gentle passive range-of-motion and inhibition techniques to decrease synergistic posturing. (Therapist will monitor and train primary service provider and family weekly, and as needed.)

3. Educational

Educational services are designed for children with a disability that affects his or her educational achievement and/or performance. Services are described under Part B of IDEA. Physical therapy is considered a related service and, as such, service provision can only be designed and rendered in a manner that enables a child to benefit from special education within the least restrictive environment. Therapeutic plans must be educationally relevant and consistent with the child's IEP (Fig. 6.2). Treatment is provided within the child's school and promotes activity-based intervention. Physical therapists serve collaboratively with team members. As educational programs move toward inclusive settings, therapists will be expected to work cooperatively with a variety of educational service personnel. Transdisciplinary teamwork and integrated service plans are becoming common. These models require therapists to spend increasing amounts of time in role releasing, monitoring programs, consulting with providers, and designing activity-based strategies, while spending possibly less time providing direct service. Table 6.4 outlines the differences between early intervention and Educational programs.

4. Private Practice

Private practice pediatric physical therapy continues to grow. Unlike the common, clinic-based, outpatient therapy practices, the private practitioner servicing children often treats children in the variety of delivery systems previously discussed.

Therapists assume responsibility to provide service under the legislative and regulatory constraints of the service delivery environment. Generally, therapists provide these services under two contractual agreements: (a) with individual children and families or (b) with a service provider (for example, local education agency, hospital, or early interven-

Child's Name: Jennifer Andersen
Birthdate: 11/6/92 **Age:** 4 months

Developmental Levels:

Fine motor	1 month	Gross Motor	<1 month
Cognitive	1–2 months	Language	2 months
Self-help	1–2 months	Social-emotional	2 months

Health and Medical Information: Jennifer was born at 28 weeks' gestation. Neonatal complications included BPD, IVH-3, apnea, and FTT. She has been home from the hospital for 1 month. Her health has been stable. She has seen her pediatrician twice since discharge. The apnea monitor is no longer necessary.

Other Information: In addition to receiving pediatric care through the ABC HMO, she is followed by the Follow-up Clinic at Teaching Hospital. Jennifer is to attend the Big Co. Child Care Center when she is 5 months old. The director, Ms. Smith, is aware that Jennifer was born prematurely.

Child's Strengths and Needs: Jennifer's developmental strengths are her sociability and her ability to hold objects when placed in her hands. She is also tolerant of interaction and is beginning to sleep for longer periods. Jennifer continues to have difficulty feeding from a bottle. It is difficult for her to maintain her head upright and reach out. Also, she prefers to stand and her legs tend to stiffen when she does stand.

Family's Strengths and Needs: Ms. Anderson and her mother are a very warm, open and loving family. They are very supportive of one another. Jennifer's father, Bill Agnew, is also very supportive of Ms. Anderson and is very involved in the care of Jennifer. They are all aware that when Ms. Anderson returns to work, a coordinated effort on their parts will be needed. They would like to work with the EIP to ensure that the services Jennifer needs are comprehensive. They continue to be concerned about Jennifer's feeding and whether it will be possible for her to be in the Child Care Center. Also, they are expressing more concern about the stiffness in Jennifer's legs and what that means.

Outcomes:
1. Ms. Anderson and Mr. Agnew would like a strategy to improve Jennifer's feeding.
2. Ms. Anderson and Mr. Agnew would like physical therapy for Jennifer.
3. Ms. Anderson would like information on alternative child care arrangements in case Jennifer cannot go to the Child Care Center.

Figure 6.1. Sample Individualized Family Service Plan (IFSP) Anywhere Early Intervention Program (EIP)

Outcome: #1
Ms. Anderson and Mr. Agnew would like a strategy to improve Jennifer's feeding skills.
Strategies/Activities:
1. The physical therapist will discuss with the nutritionist and the speech therapist strategies to improve oral-motor skills.
2. The physical therapist will instruct all caregivers in appropriate oral-motor intervention strategies.

Criteria/Time lines:
The physical therapist will make a home visit during mealtime within 5 days to initiate this service.

Outcome: #2
Ms. Anderson and Mr. Agnew would like physical therapy for Jennifer.
Strategies/Activities:
1. Physical therapy will be initiated within 5 days. Physical therapy will be given in the home initially and, if necessary, in the Child Care Center.
2. The physical therapist will provide specific activities and strategies to improve head control, decrease shoulder retraction and elevation, promote symmetrical movements of the extremities, and promote a tight seal on the nipple during feeding.

Criteria/Timelines:
The timelines are listed next to each activity. The need for therapy will be reevaluated in 6 months.

Outcome: #3
Ms. Anderson would like information on alternative child care arrangements in case Jennifer cannot go to the Child Care Center.
Strategies/Activities:
1. Ms. Kolski (service coordinator) will discuss with Ms. Smith at the Child Care Center their policy on children with special healthcare needs and what arrangements can be made.
2. Ms. Kolski will also gather information on family child-care providers and other child care centers that would accept children with special healthcare needs.

Criteria/Timelines:
Ms. Kolski will meet with Ms. Smith within the next 10 days.

Child's Name:	Jennifer Anderson	**Birthdate:**	11/6/92
Address:	1221 West Avenue, #3 Anywhere, Anyplace 01122		
Phone:	111-555-6161		

Service Coordinator: Karen Kolski, MA

Figure 6.1. continued

IFSP Team Members and Signatures:
Anne Anderson, mother
Gloria Anderson, grandmother
Bill Agnew, father
Karen Kolski, service coordinator

Frequency, Intensity, and Duration of Services:
Services will begin immediately and continue as needed until the September after Jennifer's third birthday when she is eligible for preschool. Frequency and intensity will vary; see individual outcomes.

IFSP Review Dates:	3/8/92	9/12/92
	3/12/93	9/18/93
Transition Plan:	X Not Applicable	

Parent Signature(s):

This plan represents our wishes. I (we) understand and agree with it, and I (we) authorize Anywhere Early Intervention Program to carry out this plan with me (us).

Figure 6.1. continued

tion program). Both agreements will influence the model of therapy the therapist will utilize. Table 6.6 describes factors that may influence contractual status as an employee or as an independent contractor.

Models of Service Delivery

In addition to team models of service delivery, therapists must consider (1) the focus of therapeutic services, and (2) method of delivery.

1. Focus
   a. Prevention-intervention: intervention planned to prevent or alleviate effects of biological or environmental factors on development
   b. Remedial: to improve components of movement (for example, weakness or range of motion) or to promote specific developmental skills
   c. Compensation: to minimize the effects of a disability through the use of external devices or instruction in compensatory skills to promote function
2. Method
   a. Isolated: Therapist identifies deficits and specific child's needs, designs a plan, and provides services outside child's environment (clinic, separate classroom, separate area in classroom or home); often programming designed with a remedial focus

Student's Name: Paul McCartney **DOB:** 3/10/86 **Age:** 7 years
Parent's Name: John McCartney & Ann Clemons
Address: 111 North Second Street
Andersonville, OH
School: Blair Elementary **Grade:** 1st **Diagnosis:** Cerebral Palsy
Teacher: Jeffrey Kincade

Summary of Current Level of Performance:
Cognition: WISC-III: Within normal limits
Language: Peabody Picture Vocabulary Test: 6 years, 3 months
Gross Motor: Peabody Developmental Motor Scales: 3 years, 2 months
Fine Motor: Peabody Developmental Motor Scales: 4 years
Visual-Motor: Test of Visual Motor Integration: 5 years, 6 months
Academic Achievement:

Reading: WRAT: grade level
Writing: Difficulty using a pencil
Math: WRAT: grade level

Other:
Endurance very poor; unable to walk up stairs to participate in library, music, or art. Speed of ambulation is very poor; unable to walk to gym to participate in gym class. Penmanship is illegible and he is unable to complete a number of work papers such as a spelling test.

Annual Goals:
1. Paul's language skills will be at age level
2. Paul will improve speed and endurance during walking
3. Paul will complete a spelling test in 20 minutes

Classroom placement: regular

Related services	*Model*	*Time*
Speech-Language Pathology	Consultative	30 min/week
Occupational Therapy	Integrated	60 min/week
Physical Therapy	Direct	60 min/week

Parent's Signature: **Date:**

Team Members: Teacher—Jeffrey Kincade
PT—John Wilson
OT—Karen Martins
Speech-language pathologist—Nancy Ledger

Figure 6.2. Sample of Individualized Education Plan (IEP) (section pertaining to PT only)

Physical Therapy

Annual Goal: Paul will improve speed and endurance during gait

Short Team Objectives:	*Initiation Date*	*Completion Date*	*Evaluation Criteria*
1. Given verbal instruction, Paul will ascend and descend one 12-step flight of stairs using 1 handrail and a bilateral foot placement within 5 minutes 2 times/day for 5 days	9/10/94	12/10/94	1. Time test therapist observation
2. With verbal instruction, Paul will walk a distance of 100 feet within 3 minutes for 5 consecutive days	9/10/94	12/10/94	2. Therapist observation time test

Figure 6.2. continued

b. Integrated: Services are provided in a functional context. Therapist designs treatment plans and provides services within the context that is relevant to the needs of the child. Consistent with "least restrictive environment" mandate of IDEA
c. Direct: "Hands-on" treatment. Typical for the isolated model, but is also incorporated into the integrated model to:
   - Assess child
   - Determine intervention strategies
   - Train others
   - Problem solve
   - Modify program
d. Consultation: Services are infrequent, of short duration, and by request. Therapist is not responsible for the child's outcome, but provides information and/or expertise to solve a specifically stated problem
e. Monitoring: Therapist instructs another in an intervention plan and provides ongoing support and guidance to the implementor in order to ensure successful implementation of program

Table 6.4. Differences Between the Features of Early Intervention and School Programs

Feature	Early Intervention	School
Program Model	Family-centered	Child-centered
Primary Program Focus	Promotion/Facilitation Prevention-Intervention	Remedial/Compensatory
Evaluation	Eligibility Current status	Placement IEP development
Assessment	Programming needs	(Not included)
Family Assessment	Voluntary to identify family strength, needs, and concerns related to infant	(Not included)
Services	Wide variety (medical, therapeutic, education, and psychosocial)	Instruction and related services necessary to benefit from special education
Review	Periodic (6-month and annual)	
Location of Services	Community-based	School-based
Agency Responsibility	Variable	Education
Parent Involvement	Integral team member	Passive participant
Planning Document	IFSP	IEP

DOCUMENTATION

Purpose

1. Facilitates efficacious treatment
2. Provides method of communication among therapist, family, and other service providers
3. Justifies reimbursement
4. Legal record
5. Promotes accountability

Table 6.5. Comparison of the IEP to the Individualized Family Service Plan (IFSP)

Component	IEP	IFSP
Performance	Present level of educational performance	Present level of development
Family	No provision	With agreement from family, includes a statement of the family's strengths and needs related to enhancing the development of the child
Goals	Annual goals Short-term objectives	Annual outcome
Services	Education and related services	Early intervention services
Setting	Least restrictive education environment; inclusion	Variety of inclusionary settings including the home
Medical Services	No provision	Statement of medical services necessary to meet child's needs
Timelines	Projected dates for initiation of services and the anticipated duration of services	Projected dates for initiation of services and the anticipated duration of services
Documentation	Objective criteria, evaluation procedures, and schedules for determining whether objectives are being met annually	Criteria, procedures, timelines on semi-annual basis
Service Coordinator	No provision	Name of service coordinator
Transition of Planning	No provision	Steps are outlined that will support the child, family, and team in moving from EI to preschool

General Considerations

1. The service provision setting may dictate type and frequency of documentation
2. Needs of individual children contribute to type of documentation
3. Needs, responsibility, and model of team
4. Payors of service
5. Governmental and accreditation regulations
6. Professional licensing regulations

RUMBA (developed by Quality Assurance Division of AOTA)

R—Is documentation relevant (functional)
U—Is it understandable (to family, team members)
M—Stated in measurable terms
B—Behavioral data
A—Are plans achievable

Types of Documentation Plans Based on Intervention Settings

1. Hospitals/Rehabilitation Centers
    - Problem-Oriented Medical Record (POMR)
        - SOAP
            - S—subjective
            - O—objective
            - A—assessment
            - P—plan
        - non-SOAP
            - problem, plan, results
2. Early Intervention and Educational Programs
    - Team-developed intervention plans
        - IFSP vs IEP

Figures 6.1 and 6.2 exemplify the IFSP used in early intervention and the IEP used in educational programs. Although similar in many regards, the IFSP (a) is process oriented; thus the process of collaborating with family members to develop the plan is regarded as important as the plan itself. (b) The IFSP is family centered. The IEP is (a) product oriented (focused on what child is to learn) and (b) is child-focused.

Both plans are written with all team members, including the family. All team members have an opportunity to contribute to the plan and/or outcome and to prioritize goals. Families under the IEP process are often passive participants of professionally designed plans. Families under the IFSP process are equal team members and have authority to direct the plan and establish outcomes.

Table 6.6. Factors That May Influence Employee vs. Independent Contractor Status

Employee	Independent Contractor
1. Assuming no employment contract, discharge of or resignation by individual before completion of work would not be breach of contract	1. Discharge of or resignation by individual before completion of work would be breach of contract
2. Employer furnishes the tools, materials, and/or equipment to perform the work	2. Individual furnishes his or her own tools, materials, and/or equipment, especially where it involves substantial investment
3. Services are performed on employer's premises	3. Individual is not required to work on employer's premises
4. Individual receives fixed hourly, weekly, or monthly wage	4. Individual receives a lump sum payment for work; has a possibility of sustaining a loss
5. Individual does not regularly offer his or her services to the general public	5. Individual offers services to general public, especially professional persons such as physicians, lawyers, dentists, accountants, and engineers, even though he or she may bill by the hour
6. No one else may substitute his or her services for individual's services	6. Individual is permitted to employ assistants, with exclusive right to supervise and delegate to them
7. Individual has continuing relationship with employer	7. Individual is hired to do specific job or piece of work
8. Contract is for purchase of labor	8. Contract is for purchase of product
9. Individual receives periodic or sporadic training (formally or informally) from employer	9. Individual does not receive training from employer on an ongoing basis
10. Relationship exists between services of individual and function and scope of employer's business; success of business may depend on actions of individual	10. Services performed by individual are not in the usual course of employer's business

Table 6.6. continued

Employee	Independent Contractor
11. Hours of work are established by employer	11. Individual determines when work will be done
12. Individual is required to submit regular oral or written reports to employer	12. Individual is not required to account for his or her time
13. Employer reimburses business or traveling expenses	13. Individual is responsible for his or her own business or traveling expenses
14. Individual devotes full time to business of employer	14. Individual works for more than 1 employer, who may be competitors
15. Individual is restricted from accepting other work	15. Individual may accept other work, including competitors'
16. Individual is required to comply with instructions about when, where, and how he or she is to work (this includes the *right* to require such compliance)	16. The person for whom the services are performed does not have the right to require compliance with instructions
17. Individual performs services in the order or sequence set by person for whom services are performed (this includes the *right* of the other person to set the order of sequence)	17. The person for whom the services are performed does not have the right to set the order or sequence of services
18. Lack of investment in facilities	18. Investment in facilities (special scrutiny for home offices)

Reprinted from *Physical Therapy Practice in Educational Environments,* (1990; 7.7),

3. Community-Based Posteducational Institutional Programs

IHP: The Individualized Habilitation Plan. Similar to IEP or IFSP, but primarily developed for individuals with developmental disabilities that have graduated from an educational program. Focus is on vocational program, independent living, and functional skill training.

Coding Systems

These are standardized notations to indicate the diagnosis of the client and the procedures or services provided. Three major coding systems exist.

1. ICD-9-CM: International Classification of Diseases, Ninth Revision, Clinical Modification
   a. Classifies illness, injuries, and services
   b. Provider must list principal and secondary diagnoses that indicate referral for physical therapy. Must be as specific as possible
   c. V Codes: Identifies visits with practitioners for factors influencing health status but not treatment of acute disease; for example, fitting of an orthosis or a walker
   d. Codes: Describe events surrounding an injury; for example, motor vehicle accidents
   e. The diagnostic description of the current problem should be defined by:
      - Client's subjective problem/complaint
      - Problem's date of onset
      - Objective evaluation/assessment of findings confirming diagnosis
      - Functional outcomes
2. CPT codes: Physicians Current Procedural Terminology
   a. Describes medical services and procedures
   b. Widely used by private and public insurers and managed care providers
   c. Documentation with CPT codes should describe:
      - Code name
      - Evaluation and treatment of procedure performed
      - Responses to procedure
      - Date of procedure
      - Time required to perform procedure
      - Cost
   d. Codes most often used by pediatric physical therapy include:
      - 97110—Therapeutic exercise
      - 97116—Gait training
      - 97112—Neuromuscular reeducation

3. HCPCS—Level II: Health Care Financing Administration's Common Procedure Coding System
   a. Used for billing Medicaid, Medicare, and some third-party payers
   b. Intended to supplement CPT coding system by including nonphysician services, durable medical equipment, and supplies
   c. Treatment program involving supplies and equipment should describe:
      - Therapeutic necessity for equipment
      - Substantiation for the particular piece of equipment/device
      - Therapeutic response to the equipment or device
4. DSM-IV: Diagnostic and Statistical Manual of Mental Disorders—Fourth Edition
   a. Provides classifications and descriptions of the clinical features of mental disorders. These disorders and/or disabilities are often seen by pediatric physical therapists, many in the realm of developmental disabilities (MR, ADHD, LD, etc.)
   b. All DSM-IV codes are legitimate ICD-9-CM codes
   c. Manual provides comprehensive definitions and descriptions in order to differentiate among similar diagnostic categories; decision trees are also provided for differential diagnosis

Resources

Government Agencies

Administration on Developmental Disabilities
3250-D Hubert Humphrey Building
200 Independence Avenue, SW
Washington, DC 20201
(202) 245-2890

Clearinghouse on Disability Information
400 Maryland Avenue, SW
Room 3132 Switzer Building
Washington, DC 20202
(202) 732-1241

Division of Services for Children with Special Health Needs, Bureau of Maternal Child Health
U.S. Department of Health and Human Services
5600 Fisher's Lane
Room 18A27
Rockville, MD 20857
(301) 443-2350

Head Start Bureau
U.S. Department of Health and Human Services
P.O. Box 1182
Washington, DC 20013
(202) 205-8560

Office of Special Education and Rehabilitation Services (OSERS)
U.S. Department of Education
Switzer Building
330 C Street, SW
Room 3132
Washington, DC 20202
(202) 205-8723

President's Committee on Mental Retardation
330 Independence Avenue, SW
Washington, DC 20201
(202) 732-1294

Professional Organizations

Academy of Dentistry for the Handicapped
211 East Chicago Avenue
Chicago, IL 60611

American Academy for Cerebral Palsy and Developmental Medicine (AACPDM)
6300 N. River Road
Rosemount, IL 60018
(708) 698-1635

American Occupational Therapy Association (AOTA)
4720 Montgomery Lane
Bethesda, MD 20816
(301) 652-2682

American Physical Therapy Association (APTA)
1111 N. Fairfax Street
Alexandria, VA 22314
(703) 684-2782
(800) 999-2782

American Speech-Language-Hearing Association (ASHA)
10801 Rockville Pike
Rockville, MD 20852-3279
(301) 897-5700
(800) 638-8255

Association for the Care of Children's Health (ACCH)
3615 Wisconsin Avenue, NW
Washington, DC 20016
(202) 244-1801

Council for Exceptional Children (CEC)
1920 Association Drive
Reston, VA 22091
(703) 620-3660
(800) 328-0272

Neuro-Developmental Treatment Association (NDTA)
P.O. Box 14613
Chicago, IL 60614

RESNA
1101 Connecticut Avenue, NW
Suite 700
Washington, DC 20036
(202) 857-1140

Sensory Integration Internation (SII)
1602 Cabrillo Avenue
Torrance, CA 90501
(310) 320-9986

The Association for Severe Handicaps (TASH)
11201 Greenwood Avenue, North
Seattle, WA 98133
(206) 361-8870

The Commission on the Mental and Physical Disability Law, American Bar Association
1800 M Street, NW
Washington, DC 20036
(202) 331-2240

Advocacy

American Council for the Blind
1010 Vermont Avenue, NW
Suite 1100
Washington, DC 20005
(202) 393-3666
(800) 242-8666

Disability Rights Education Defense Fund
2212 6th Street
Berkeley, CA 94710
(510) 644-2555
(800) 466-4232

Kids on the Block
9385 C Gerwig Lane
Columbia, MD 21046
(301) 290-9095
(800) 368-KIDS

Learning Disabilities Association of America
4156 Library Road
Pittsburgh, PA 15234
(412) 341-1515

National Association of Developmental Disabilities Council (NADDC)
1234 Massachusetts Avenue, NW
Suite 203
Washington, DC 20005
(202) 347-1234

National Association of the Deaf
814 Thayer Avenue
Silver Spring, MD 20910
(310) 587-1788

The ARC (formerly Association for Retarded Citizens) National Organization on Mental Retardation
500 E. Border Street
Suite 300
Arlington, TX 76011
(817) 261-6003
(800) 433-5255

Parent Support Groups

Estate Planning for Persons with Disabilities
3100 Arapahoe Avenue
Suite 112
Boulder, CO 80303
(800) 448-1071

International Institute for the Visually Impaired
230 Central Street
Auburndale, MA 02166
(617) 332-4014

Life Services for the Handicapped
352 Park Avenue
Suite 703
New York, NY 10010
(212) 532-6740

National Association of Private Schools for Exceptional Children
1522 K Street, NW
Suite 1032
Washington, DC 20005
(202) 408-3338

National Down Syndrome Congress
1605 Chantilly Drive
Suite 250
Atlanta, GA 30324
(800) 232-NDSC
(404) 633-1555

National Lekotek Center
2100 Ridge Avenue
Evanston, IL 60201
(708) 328-0001
(800) 366-PLAY

Parents of Premature and High Risk Infants International, Inc.
33 West 42nd Street
New York, NY 10036
(212) 840-1259

Disability Specific Organizations

American Brittle Bone Society (ABBS)
1256 Merrill Drive
West Chester, PA 19380
(215) 692-6248

American Juvenile Arthritis Organization
1314 Spring Street, NW
Atlanta, GA 30309
(404) 872-7100

Association for Children with Down Syndrome, Inc (ACDS)
2616 Martin Avenue
Bellmore, NY 11710
(516) 221-4700

Autism Society of America
7910 Woodmont Avenue #650
Bethesda, MD 20814
(800) 328-8476

AVENUES, National Support Group for Arthrogryposis Multiplex Congenita
P.O. Box 5192
Sonora, CA 95370
(209) 928-3689

Cleft Palate Foundation
1218 Grandview Avenue
Pittsburgh, PA 15211
(800) 24-CLEFT
(412) 481-1376

Cystic Fibrosis Foundation
6931 Arlington Road
Bethesda, MD 20814
(301) 951-4422
(800) FIGHT CF

Foundation for Children with Learning Disabilities
Grand Central Station
P.O. Box 2929
New York, NY 10163
(212) 687-7211

Fragile X Foundation
P.O. Box 300233
Denver, CO 80203
(800) 835-2246 ext. 58

Learning Disabilities Association of America (LDA)
4156 Library Road
Pittsburgh, PA 15234
(412) 341-1515

Little People of America
P.O. Box 9897
Washington, DC 20016
(301) 589-0730

March of Dimes Birth Defects Foundation
1275 Mamaroneck Avenue
White Plains, NY 10605
(914) 428-7100

Muscular Dystrophy Association
810 Seventh Avenue
New York, NY 10019
(212) 586-0808

National Hemophilia Foundation
The Soho Building
110 Greene Street
Suite 303
New York, NY 10012
(212) 219-8180

Osteogenesis Imperfecta Foundation, Inc.
P.O. Box 14807
Tampa, FL 34629
(813) 855-7077

Prader-Willi Syndrome Association
2510 South Brentwood Boulevard
St. Louis, MO 63144
(314) 962-7644
(800) 926-4797

Sickle Cell Disease Association of America
3345 Wilshire Boulevard
Suite 1106
Los Angeles, CA 20010
(800) 421-8453
(213) 736-5455

Spina Bifida Association of America
4590 MacArthur Boulevard NW
Washington, DC 20007
(202) 944-3285
(800) 621-3141

Turner's Syndrome Society
York University Administrative Studies
Building #006
4700 Keele Street
Downsview, Ontario M3JIP3
Canada
(416) 736-5023

National Organizations

Joseph P. Kennedy Foundation
1350 New York Avenue, NW
Suite 500
Washington, DC 20005
(202) 393-1250

National Association for Down's Syndrome
P.O. Box 4542
Oak Brook, IL 60521
(708) 325-9112

National Association for Visually Handicapped
22 West 21st Street
New York, NY 10010
(212) 889-3141

or

3201 Balboa Street
San Francisco, CA 94121
(415) 221-8753
(415) 221-3201

National Braille Press
88 St. Stephen Street
Boston, MA 02115
(617) 266-6160

National Down Syndrome Society
666 Broadway
New York, NY 10012
(800) 221-4602
(212) 460-9330

National Easter Seal Society
230 West Monroe Street
Suite 1800
Chicago, IL 60606
(312) 726-6200

National Head Start Association
201-N Union Street
Suite 320
Alexandria, VA 22314
(703) 739-0875

Sibling Information Network
The University of Connecticut
Department of Educational Psychology
249 Glenbrook Road
Box U-64
Storrs, CT 06268
(203) 486-4031
(203) 486-5035

Siblings for Significant Change
105 E. 22nd Street
Room 710
New York, NY 10010
(212) 420-0776
(800) 841-8251

Specialnet
GET Education Services, Inc.
2021 K Street, NW
Suite 215
Washington, DC 20006

United Cerebral Palsy Association; UCP Research and Education Foundation
1522 K Street, NW
Suite 1112
Washington, DC 20005
(202) 842-1266
(800) 872-5827

Activity Organizations

American Association of the Deaf
3916 Lantern Drive
Silver Spring, MD 20902
(301) 585-5400

American Blind Bowlers Association
150 N. Bellaire
Louisville, KY 40206

Blind Outdoor Leisure Development, Inc. (BOLD)
533 Main Street
Aspen, CO 81611

Braille Sports Foundation
730 Hennepin Avenue
Room 301
Minneapolis, MN 55402

International Committee of Silent Sports
Gallaudet University
800 Florida Avenue NE
Washington, DC 20002
(202) 651-5000

International Council on Therapeutic Ice Skating
P.O. Box 13
State College, PA 16801

National Sports Center for the Disabled
P.O. Box 36
Winter Park, CO 80482
(303) 726-5514 ext. 179

National Wheelchair Athletic Association
4024 62nd Street
Woodside, NY 11377
(718) 424-2929

National Wheelchair Basketball Association
110 Seaton Building
University of Kentucky
Lexington, KY 40506
(606) 276-2136

North American Riding for the Handicapped Association
P.O. Box 33150
Denver, CO 80233
(800) 369-7433

Ski for Light, Inc.
1455 W. Lake Street
Minneapolis, MN 55408
(612) 827-3232

Special Olympics
1350 New York Avenue, NW
Washington, DC 20002
(202) 628-3630

Sports for the Physically Disabled
333 River Road
Ottawa, Ontario
CANADA
K1L 8B9

The American Camping Association
5000 State Road 67 North
Martinsville, IN 46151
(317) 342-8456

U.S. Association for Blind Athletes
55 W. California Avenue
Beach Haven Park, NJ 08008

U.S. Blind Golfer's Association
225 Baronne Street
28th Floor
New Orleans, LA 70112

World Games for the Deaf Committee
1500 N. Coalter Street, B-6
Staunton, VA 24401

Clearinghouse/ Educational Information

American Foundation for the Blind
15 West 16th Street
New York, NY 10011
(212) 620-2147
(800) 232-5463

American Society for Deaf Children
East 10th and Tahlequah Streets
Sulphur, OK 73086
(800) 942-ASDC

Americans with Disabilities Act Information Line
U.S. Department of Justice
Civil Rights Division
P.O. Box 66118
Washington, DC 20035-6118
(202) 514-0301

Clearinghouse on Disability Information Office of Special Education and Rehabilitative Services
U.S. Department of Special Education
Switzer Building
400 Maryland Avenue
Room 3132
Washington, DC 20202
(202) 732-1241

Disabled Children's Computer Group
Fairmont School
724 Kearney Street
El Cerrito, CA 94530
(510) 525-5235

Epilepsy Foundation of America, Children, Youth and Families
4351 Garden City Drive
Suite 406
Landover, MD 20785
(301) 459-3701
(800) 332-1000 - for information and referral
(800) 332-4050 - for professional/technical library

HEATH Resource Center
Higher Education and Adult Education for People with Handicaps National Clearinghouse
One Dupont Circle, NW
Suite 800
Washington, DC 20036
(202) 939-9320
(800) 544-3284

IBM National Support Center for Persons with Disabilities
P.O. Box 2150
Atlanta, GA 30055
(800) IBM-2133

National Center for Education in Maternal and Child Health (NCEMCH)
2000 15th Street, N
Suite 701
Arlington, VA 22201-2617
(703) 524-7802

National Center on Postsecondary Transition for Students with Learning Disabilities
Learning Disability College Unit
University of Connecticut
East Hartford, CT 06108
(203) 486-2000

National Information Center for Children and Youth with Handicaps (NICHY)
Box 1492
Washington, DC 20036
(800) 999-5599
(703) 522-0870

National Library Service for the Blind and Physically Handicapped
Library of Congress
1291 Taylor Street, NW
Washington, DC 20542
(202) 287-5100

National Organization for Rare Disorders
100 Route 37
P.O. Box 8923
New Fairfield, CT 06812
(800) 447-6673
(203) 746-6518

National Rehabilitation Information Center and Able Data
c/o MACRO Systems
8455 Colesville Road
Suite 935
Silver Spring, MD 20910
(301) 588-9284
(800) 346-2742

Equipment Suppliers—Treatment

Achievement Products
P.O. Box 9033
Canton, OH 44711
(716) 298-4700
(800) 373-4699

Alimed, Inc.
297 High Street
Dedham, MA 02026
(800) 229-2900

Ball Dynamics International
P.O. Box 24555
Denver, CO 80224
(303) 752-2255

Best Priced Products, Inc.
P.O. Box 1174
White Plains, NY 10602
(800) 824-2939

Consumer Care' Products
P.O. Box 684
810 N Water Street
Sheboygan, WI 53082
(414) 459-8353
(800) 255-7317

Danmar Products, Inc.
221 Jackson Industrial Drive
Ann Arbor, MI 48103
(800) 783-1998

Equipment Shop
P.O. Box 22
Bedford, MA 01730
(617) 275-7681

Flaghouse
150 N. MacQueston Parkway
Suite 90266
Mt. Vernon, NY 10550
(800) 221-5185

Fred Sammons, Inc.
Box 32
Brookfield, IL 60513
or
145 Tower Drive
Burr Ridge, IL 60521
(800) 323-5547

GE Miller, Inc.
540 Nepperhan Avenue
Yonkers, NY 10701
(800) 431-2924

JA Preston Corp.
60 Page Road
Clifton, NJ 07012
(201) 777-2700
(800) 631-7277

Jeasana Ltd.
P.O. Box 17
Irvington, NY 10533
(800) 443-4728

Kapable Kids
P.O. Box 250
Bohemia, NY 11716
(800) 356-1564

Kaye Products
535 Dimmocks Mill Road
Hillsborough, NC 27278
(919) 732-6444

Rifton for People with Disabilities
Route 213
Rifton, NY 12471
(914) 658-3141

Southpaw Enterprises
800 West Third Street
Dayton, OH 45407
(800) 228-1698

Sportime
One Sportime Way
Atlanta, GA 30340
(404) 449-5700

Sunrise Medical
2355 Crenshaw Boulevard
Suite 150
Torrance, CA 90501
(216) 366-5611
(800) 421-3349

TherAdapt Products, Inc.
17 West 163 Oak Lane
Bensenville, IL 60106
(708) 834-2461

Therapeutic Design, Inc.
1850 Lee Road
Winter Park, FL 32789
(407) 740-7874

Troll Learn and Play
100 Corporate Drive
Mahwah, NJ 07430
(800) 247-6106

Braces and Orthotics Materials

Alimed, Inc.
297 High Street
Dedham MA 02026
(800) 225-2610

Fred Sammons Orthopedic Catalog
Box 32
Brookfield, IL 60513
(800) 323-7305

North Coast Medical
187 Stauffer Boulevard
San Jose, CA 95125
(800) 821-9319

Smith, Nephew and Rolyan
WFR Aquaplast Corp.
One Quality Drive
P.O. Box 578
Germantown, WI 53022
(800) 228-3693

Tri-Wall Containers Company
2626 County Road 71
Butler, IN 46721
(219) 868-2151

Seating Systems

Amigo Mobility
6693 Dixie Highway
Bridgeport, MI 48722
(517) 777-2060

Best Priced Products, Inc.
P.O. Box 1174
White Plains, NY 10602
(800) 824-2939

Canadian Posture and Seating Centre, Inc.
Box 1473
Station C
Kitchner, Ontario,
Canada N2G 4P2

Canadian Wheelchair MFG, LTD
1360 Blundell Road
Mississauga, Ontario
Canada L4Y1M5

ETAC USE, Inc.
2325 Parklawn Drive
Suite P
Waukesha, WI 53186
(800) 678-3822

Everest and Jennings
3233 East Mission Oaks Boulevard
Camarillo, CA 93010
(800) 788-3633

Fortress, Inc.
827 Jefferson Avenue
Clovis, CA 93612

Gadabout Wheelchairs
1165 Portland Avenue
Rochester, NY 10533
(716) 338-2110

Sunrise Medical Co.
(Guardian Products)
12800 Wentworth
Arleta, CA 91331
(818) 982-8062

Gunnell, Inc.
8440 State Street
Millington, MI 48746
(800) 551-0055

Invacare Corp.
899 Cleveland Street
Elyria, OH 44036
(216) 329-6000

Jay Medical, LTD
P.O. Box 18656
Boulder, CO 80301
(800) 648-8282

Kid-Kart Inc.
126 Rosebud
Belgrade, MT 59714
(800) 388-5278

Mulholland Positioning Systems, Inc.
215 N. 12th Street
P.O. Box 391
Santa Paula, CA 93060
(805) 525-7165

Ortho-Kinetics, Inc.
P.O. Box 1647
Waukesha, WI 53187
(800) 558-7786

Otto Bock Orthopedic Industry, Inc.
3000 Xenium Lane, North
Minneapolis, MN 55441
(800) 328-4058

Pin Dot Products
6001 Gross Point Road
Niles, IL 60648
(708) 509-2800

Quickie Designs, Inc.
2842 Business Park Avenue
Fresno, CA 93727
(209) 292-2171

Roho, Inc.
100 Florida Avenue
Belleville, IL 62222
(618) 277-9150

Scott Designs
7085 Vaughn Avenue
Suite C
Livermore, CA 94550
(510) 294-1700

Snug Seat, Inc.
P.O. Box 1141
Matthews, NC 28106
(704) 847-0772

Sunrise Medical
2355 Crenshaw Boulevard
Suite 150
Torrance, CA 90501
(216) 366-5611
(800) 421-3349

Wheel Ring, Inc.
199 Forest Street
Manchester, CT 06040
(203) 647-8596

Independent Living

Adaptability
P.O. Box 515
Colchester, CT 06415
(800) 243-9232

Cleo Inc.
3957 Mayfield Road
Cleveland, OH 44121
(216) 382-9700

Fred Sammons, Inc.
Box 32
Brookfield, IL 60513
or
145 Tower Drive
Burr Ridge, IL 60521
(800) 323-5547

Home Care Products, Inc.
P.O. Box 58977
Seattle, WA 98138
(206) 320-4848

Clothing

Adrian's Closet
P.O. Box 9506
Rancho Santa Fe, CA 92067
(800) 831-2577

Brace Mates
P.O. Box 58
Jackson, GA 30233
(404) 412-7793

Exceptionally Yours
60 Joseph Road
P.O. Box 3246
Framingham, MA 01701
(508) 877-9757

Independent Clothing
P.O. Box 81
Sun Prairie, WI 53590
(608) 837-2570

Plum Enterprises, Inc.
9 Clyston Circle
P.O. Box 283
Worcester, PA 19490
(800) 321-PLUM

Sister Kenny Institute
Public Relations Department
800 East 28th Street at Chicago Avenue
Minneapolis, MN 55407
(612) 863-4400 or (4630) or (4205)

Special Clothes
P.O. Box 4220
Alexandria, VA 22303
(703) 683-7343

Toys

Andeles Toys, Inc.
9 Capper Drive
Dailey Industrial Park
Pacific, MO 63069

Hals Pals
P.O. Box 3490
Winter Park, CO 80482

Jeasana Ltd.
P.O. Box 17
Irvington, NY 10533
(800) 443-4728

Nintendo Hands Free Controller
Toys for Special Children
385 Warburton Avenue
Hastings, NY 10706
(800) 422-2602
(914) 478-0960

Toys for Special Children
Steven Kanor
8 Main Street
Hastings on the Hudson, NY 10706
(800) 832-8697

Triad, Inc.
P.O. Box 1364
Cumberland, MD 21502
(301) 759-2707

Troll Learn and Play
100 Corporate Drive
Mahwah, NJ 07430
(800) 247-6106

Communication/Technology

Apple Computer, Inc.
Apple Office of Special Education
20525 Mariani Avenue
Mail Stop 23 D
Cupertino, CA 95014
(800) 538-9696
(800) 776-2333 #4
(408) 996-1010

Askia Learning Products
P.O. Box 11538
Atlanta, GA 30310
(800) 635-3046

Communication Aids for Children and Adults
c/o Creastwood Company
6625 N. Sidney Place
Department 127
Milwaukee, WI 53209
(414) 352-5678

Communication Skill Builders
3830 East Bellvue
P.O. Box 42050
Tucson, AZ 85733
(520) 323-7500

IBM Corporation
IBM National Support Center for Persons with Disabilities
Box C-1030
Atlanta, GA 30055
(800) 426-3333

LC Technologies
4415 Glenn Rose Street
Fairfax, VA 22032
(800) 733-5284

Prentke Romich
1022 Heyl Road
Wooster, OH 44691
(800) 262-1984

Salco
11445 150th Street, East
Nerstrand, MN 55053
(507) 645-8720

Sources

Chapter 1. Growth and Development

Bacon GE, Spenser ML, Hopwood NJ, Kelch RP. Pediatric endocrinology. Chicago: Year Book Medical Publishers, 1990.

Bekoff A. Embryonic motor output and movement patterns: Relationship to postnatal behavior. In: SmothermanWP, Robinson SR, eds. Behavior of the fetus. Caldwell, New Jersey: Telford Press, 1988.

Bottos M, Dalla Barba B, Stephani D, et al. Locomotor strategies preceding independent walking: Prospective study of neurological and language development in 424 cases. Developmental Medicine and Child Neurology, 1989;31:25–34.

Cintas HM. Fetal movements: An overview. Physical and Occupational Therapy in Pediatrics, 1987;7:1–15.

Cole M, Cole S. The development of children. New York: Scientific American Books, 1989.

Dahlmann N, Petersen K. Influences of environmental conditions during infancy on final body stature. Pediatric Research 1977;11;695–700.

Fung YC. Biomechanics. New York: Springer-Verlag, 1990.

Graham JM, Smith's recognizable patterns of human deformation. 2nd ed., Philadelphia: W.B. Saunders, 1988.

Hall JG, Froster-Iskenius UG, Allanson JE. Handbook of normal physical measurements. Oxford: Oxford University Press, 1989.

Hamill PVV, Drizd PA, Johnson CL, Reed RB, Roche R. National Center for Health Statistics (NCHS) growth curves for children, birth to eighteen years. DHEW Publication no. (PHS) 78–1650. Washington, DC: U.S. Government Printing Office, 1977.

Harris SR, Osborn JA, Weinberg J, Loock C, Junaid K. Effects of prenatal alcohol exposure on neuromotor and cognitive development during early childhood: A series of case reports. Physical Therapy 1993;73:609–617.

Hensinger RN. Standards in pediatric orthopedics. New York: Raven Press, 1986.

Hill RM, Hegemier S, Tennyson LM. The fetal alcohol syndrome: A multihandicapped child. NeuroToxicology 1989; 10:585–596.

Jones KL, Smith's recognizable patterns of human malformation. 4th ed. Philadelphia: W.B. Saunders, 1988.

Kaltenbach KA, Finnegan LP. Prenatal narcotic exposure: Prenatal and developmental effects. NeuroToxicology 1989;10:597–604.

Lampl M, Veldhuis JD, Johnson ML. Saltation and stasis: A model of human growth. Science 1992;258:801–803.

McKusick VA: Mendelian inheritance in man: Catalogs of autosomal dominants, autosomal recessives, and X-linked phenotypes, 9th ed. Baltimore: Johns Hopkins University Press, 1990.

Moore KL, Persaud TVN. The developing human, 5th ed. Philadelphia: WB Saunders, 1993.

Osborne JA, Harris SR, Weinberg J. Fetal alcohol syndrome: Review of the literature with implications for physical therapists. Physical Therapy 1993;73: 599–607.

Sparling J, ed. Concepts in fetal movement research. Physical and Occupational Therapy 1992;12(2,3):1–234.

Thompson MW, McInnes RR, Willard HF. Thompson and Thompson: Genetics in medicine, 5th ed. Philadelphia: WB Saunders, 1991.

Van Sant A. The child with orthopedic problems. In: Peyton O, ed. Manual of physical therapy. New York: Churchill Livingstone, 1989: 495–541.

Wiedemann HR, Kunze J, Dibbern H. Atlas of clinical syndromes. 2nd ed. St. Louis: Mosby, 1992.

Chapter 2. Measurement

Campbell SK. Using standardized tests in clinical practice. Alexandria, VA: American Physical Therapy Association, 1990. In Touch Series; Topics in Pediatrics.

Duncan PW, Weiner DK, Chandler J, et al. Functional reach: A new measure of balance. J Gerontal Med Sci 1990;45: 192–197.

Gibbs ED, Teti DM, eds. Interdisciplinary assessment of infants: a guide for early intervention professionals. Baltimore, MD: Paul H. Brookes Publishing Co., 1990.

King-Thomas L, Hacker BJ, eds. A therapist's guide to pediatric assessment. Boston: Little, Brown & Co., 1987.

Thomas CC. Reflex testing: Methods for the evaluation of central nervous system development. 2nd ed. Springfield, IL: Charles C. Thomas, 1973.

Wilhelm IJ. Physical therapy assessment in early infancy. New York: Churchill Livingstone, 1993.

Wilson JM. Cerebral palsy. In: Campbell SK, ed. Pediatric neurologic physical therapy. New York, NY: Churchill Livingstone, 1991;301–360.

Chapter 3. Pediatric Disorders

Campbell SK. Physical therapy for children. Philadelphia: WB Saunders, 1994.

Carmick J. Clinical use of neuromuscular electrical stimulation for children with cerebral palsy. Physical Therapy 1993; 73:505–527.

Castaneda AR, Jonas RA, Mayer JE, Hanley FL. Cardiac surgery of the neonate and infant. Philadelphia: WB Saunders, 1994.

Coster WJ, Haley SM. Conceptualization and measurement of disablement in infants and young children. Infants and Young Children 1992;4:11–22.

Dunn JM, Donner RM. Heart transplant in children. Mount Kisko, NY: Futura Publishing Co., 1990.

Eckersley P. Elements of paediatric physiotherapy. Edinborough: Churchill Livingstone, 1993.

Guccione AA. Physical therapy diagnosis and the relationship between impairments and function. Physical Therapy 1991;71:499–504.

Hylton NM. Postural and functional impact of dynamic AFOs and FOs in a pediatric population. Journal of Prosthetics and Orthotics 1989; 2:40–53.

Jones KL. Smith's recognizable patterns of human malformation. Philadelphia: WB Saunders, 1988.

Krebs D. ed. Prehension assessment: Prosthetic therapy for the upper-limb child amputee. Thorofare, NJ: Thomas Slack, 1987.

Milunsky A, Jick H, Jick SS, Bruell CL, MacLaughlin DS, Rothman KJ, Willett W. Multivitamin/folic acid supplementation in early pregnancy reduces the prevalence of neural tube defects. Journal of American Medical Association 1989;262:2847–2852.

Nagi SZ. Disability concepts revisited: Implications for prevention. In: Pope AM, Tarlov DC, eds. Disability in America. Washington, DC: National Academy Press, 1991:309–327.

O'Leary JA. Shoulder dystocia and birth injury. New York: McGraw-Hill, 1992.

Sandford MK, Kissling GE, Joubert PE. Neural tube defect etiology: New evidence concerning maternal hyperthermia, health and diet. Developmental Medicine and Child Neurology 1992; 34:661–675.

Tecklin JS, ed. Pediatric physical therapy. 2nd ed. Philadelphia: JB Lippincott, 1994.

Wenger DR, Rang M. The art and practice of children's orthopedics. New York: Raven Press, 1993.

Wood PHN. The language of disablement: A glossary relating to disease and its consequences. International Rehabilitation Medicine 1980;2:86–92.

World Health Organization. International Classification of Impairments, Disabilities, and Handicaps. Geneva: World Health Organization, 1980.

Chapter 4. Pediatric Equipment

Bergen AF, Presperin J, Tullman T. Positioning for function: wheelchairs and other assistive technology. Valhalla, NY: Valhalla Rehabilitation Publications, Inc., 1990.

Church G, Glennen S. The handbook of assistive technology. San Diego, CA: Singular Publishing Group, Inc., 1992.

Donatelli R. The biomechanics of the foot and ankle. Philadelphia, PA: FA Davis, 1990.

Tecklin JS, ed. Pediatric physical therapy. 2nd ed. Philadelphia, PA: JB Lippincott, 1994.

Trelfar E, Hobson D, Taylor S, Monahan L, Shaw CG. Seating and mobility: for persons with physical disabilities. Tucson, AZ: Therapy Skill Builders, 1993.

Chapter 5. Locomotion

Abitbol MM. Quadrupedalism and the acquisition of bipedalism in human children. Gait and Posture 1993; 1:189–195.

Beck RJ, Andriacci TP, Kuo KN, et al. Changes in the gait patterns of growing children. Journal of Bone and Joint Surgery 1981;63A (9):1452–1456.

Benson JB. Season of birth and onset of locomotion: Theoretical and methodological implications. Infant Behavior and Development 1993;16:69–81.

Bottos M, Dalla Barba B, Stefani D, et al: Locomotor strategies preceding independent walking: Prospective study of neurological and language development in 424 cases. Developmental Medicine and Child Neurology 1989;31:25–34.

Cintas HM. The accomplishment of walking: Aspects of the ascent. Pediatric Physical Therapy 5:61–68, 1993.

Cintas HM. Cross-cultural similarities and differences in development and the impact of parental expectations on motor behavior. Pediatric Physical Therapy (In Press). 1995.

Cintas HM. Cross-cultural variation in infant motor development. Physical and Occupational Therapy in Pediatrics 8:1–20, 1988.

Fung YC. Biomechanics. New York: Springer-Verlag, 1990:1.

Gage JR. Gait analysis in cerebral palsy. Clinics in Developmental Medicine No. 121. London: Mac Keith Press, 1991.

Jones KL. Smith's recognizable patterns of human malformation, 4th ed. Philadelphia: WB Saunders, 1988.

Kucera M, Macek M, Javurek J. A method for estimation of the changes in bipedal locomotion. In: Berg K, Eriksson BO, eds. Children and Exercise IX. 1980; 49–52.

Lee DN, Aronson E. Visual proprioceptive control of standing in human infants. Perception and Psychophysics 15: 529–532. Cited in Woolacott et al., 1989, p. 82.

Largo RH, Molinari L, Weber M, et al: Early development of locomotion, significance of prematurity, cerebral palsy and sex. Developmental Medicine and Child Neurology 1985;27:183–191.

McCabe ME. Qualitative analysis of normal fetal movement patterns at 17–18 weeks' gestation. Master's thesis and videotape documentation. Madison, WI: University of Wisconsin-Madison, 1984.

Myklebust BM. A review of myotatic reflexes and the development of motor control and gait in infants and children: a special communication. Physical Therapy 1990;70:188–203.

Perry J. Gait analysis: normal and pathological function. Thorofare, NJ: Stack, 1992.

Rose J, Gamble JG. Human walking, 2nd ed. Baltimore: Williams & Wilkins, 1994.

Sparrow WA: Creeping patterns of human adults and infants. American Journal of Physical Anthropology 1989;78: 387–401.

Sutherland DH, Valencia F. Pediatric gait: Normal and abnormal development. In: Drennen JC, ed. The child's foot and ankle. New York: Raven, 1992, pp. 19–35.

Sutherland DH, Olshen RA, Biden EN, Wyatt MP. The development of mature walking. Clinics in Developmental Medicine No. 104/105. London: Mac Keith Press. 1988.

Sutherland DH, Olshen R, Cooper L, et al: The development of mature gait. Journal of Bone and Joint Surgery (Am) 1980; 62:336–353.

Thelen E, Ulrich B, Jensen J. The developmental origins of locomotion. In: Woollacott M, Shumway-Cook A, eds. The development of posture and gait across the lifespan. Columbia, SC: The University of South Carolina Press; 1989: 25–47.

Thelen E, Fisher DM. Newborn stepping: an explanation for a disappearing reflex. Developmental Psychology 1982; 18: 760–775.

Todd FN, Lamoreux LW, Skinner SR, et al. Variations in the gait of normal children. Journal of Bone and Joint Surgery 1989;71:196–204.

Wenger DR, Rang M. The art and practice of children's orthopedics. New York: Raven Press, 1993.

Winter DA. Biomechanics of human movement. New York: Wiley, 1979, Chapter 4.

Whittle MW. Gait analysis: an introduction. Oxford: Butterworth-Heinemann, 1991.

Woolacott MH, Shumway-Cook A. Development of posture and gait across the lifespan. Columbia, SC: University of South Carolina Press, 1989.

Woolacott MH, Shumway-Cook A, Williams HG. The development of posture and balance control in children. In: Woolacott MH, Shumway-Cook A. Development of posture and gait across the lifespan. Columbia, SC: University of South Carolina Press, 1989, pp. 77–96.

Zelazo PR. "Learning to Walk": recognition of higher order influences? In: Lipsitt L, Rovee C, eds. Advances in infancy research. Norwood, NJ: Ablex, 1984;3:251–256.

Chapter 6. Administrative Issues

American Physical Therapy Association. Coding and payment guide for the physical therapist. Alexandria, VA: St. Anthony Publishing, Inc., 1993.

American Physical Therapy Association. Physical therapy practice in educational environments: policies and guidelines. Alexandria, VA: American Physical Therapy Association, 1990.

Dunn W. Pediatric occupational therapy: Facilitating effective service provision. Thorofare, NJ: Slack, Inc., 1991.

Hylton J, Reed P, Hall S, Cicerillo, M. The role of the physical therapist and the occupational therapist in the school setting. Portland, OR: University Affiliated Program, Oregon Health Sciences University, 1987.

McGonigel MJ, Kaufmann RK, Johnson B. Guidelines and recommended practices for the individualized family service plan, 2nd ed. Bethesda, MD: Association for the Care of Children's Health, 1991.

Glossary

absence seizure (petit mal seizure)—loss of consciousness that lasts several seconds and is characterized by a blank, "fixed" facial expression sometimes accompanied by repeated blinking or other small, facial, muscle movements

achondroplasia—condition characterized by short limbs due to lack of cartilage formation at epiphyses of long bones

acute lymphocytic (or lymphoblastic) leukemia (ALL)—the most common childhood malignancy; usually diagnosed between 2–8 years of age. ALL is characterized by replacement of normal cells by leukemic cells in the bone marrow; these cells then spread to various organs and sites; progression is rapid.

adaptive equipment—devices used to improve function and mobility, such as walkers, wheelchairs, standers, weighted spoons, etc.

adaptive response—appropriate/functional response to an environmental demand

air splint—plastic, inflatable splint which surrounds extremity or joint to provide deep pressure or passive stretch to soft tissues or maintain joint position

alcohol block (see nerve block)

alternative communication—communication system that employs various strategies or devices to substitute for speech (for example, sign language, picture boards, word boards, etc.)

amblyopia—reduced or dimmed vision in absence of pathological condition

ankylosis—immobile, fixed state of joint; can be fibrous or bony

antigravity extension—ability to move and hold body in extended position against gravity

antigravity flexion—ability to move and hold body in flexed position against gravity

Apgar—scoring scale used to assess neonate's physical condition at 1, 5, and occasionally 10 minutes after birth; areas scored include respiratory effort, color, cry, muscle tone, and heart rate; acceptable score is between 7–10, as 2 points are possible for each of above areas

aphasia—absence or impairment of ability to speak or use signs or words to communicate

apnea—cessation of breathing; short periods of apnea common in premature infants

apnea monitor—electronic monitoring device for apneic episodes; alerts caregivers so that appropriate resuscitative measures may be taken, if necessary

appropriate for gestational age (AGA)—an infant's weight at birth which falls between the 10th and 90th percentile for that infant's gestational age

apraxia—inability to plan or perform sequenced movements

arena assessment—developmental assessment where several disciplines simultaneously assess child's skills; one team member acts as facilitator with child

Arnold-Chiari malformation (also known as **Chiari II**)—condition involving protrusion of parts of cerebellum and medulla through foramen magnum into spinal canal; associated with hydrocephalus and myelomeningocele

arthrodesis—surgical immobilization/fixation of joint for purposes of joint stabilization or reduction of a deformity

arthrogryposis multiplex congenita—condition characterized by multiple congenital joint deformations in flexed positions; intelligence generally unaffected; often includes dislocated hips and club feet

aspiration—inhalation of foreign matter into the lungs (liquid or solid); term also denotes suctioning of matter from the body

astigmatism—variation in the curvature of the eye that leads to diminished focusing ability

ataxia—impaired motor coordination during active movement due to cerebellar damage; frequently apparent in unsteady, uncoordinated, and wide-based gait

atelectasis—collapse of alveoli of the lungs

athetosis—uncontrollable, involuntary movements of the extremities

atonia—lack of muscle tone; flaccidity

"at-risk"—classification of developmental status; child is predisposed to developmental delays or future learning problems due to pregnancy, birth, or neonatal period risk factors such as prematurity, neonatal complications, medical conditions, environmental factors, exposure to teratogens, etc.

attention deficit hyperactivity disorder (ADHD)—disorder characterized by varying degrees of developmentally inappropriate inattention, impulsiveness, and hyperactivity; may also occur without hyperactivity and is then referred to as **attention deficit disorder (ADD)**

augmentative communication—methods employing various techniques or devices to supplement a person's expressive language skills which often use pictures and computer interfaces

autism—severe communication disorder accompanied by apparent lack of social interaction and varied play skills; frequently associated with self-stimulatory behaviors such as hand-flapping, rocking, or spinning; onset during infancy or childhood; most severe form of **pervasive developmental disorder (PDD)**

avascular necrosis—death of tissue or bone due to poor blood supply or vasculature in the area

axillary suspension—act of holding a child by the trunk under the arms; provides information about muscle tone ("slip-through" associated with hypotonia)

Azidothymidine (AZT)—drug used to treat HIV

babbling—repetition of consonant-vowel combinations such as "ba-ba"

BAER (brainstem auditory evoked response)—hearing test performed with scalp electrodes to detect responses within the brain to auditory stimuli; useful for babies or nonverbal children; sedation may be used during the test

Barlow (dislocation) test—technique used to determine hip dislocation; positive if the femur pistons in the acetabulum in a position of flexion and adduction

bilateral integration—ability to use both sides of the body in a functionally interactive manner, for example, threading a needle or stringing a bead

brachial plexus injury—damage to the peripheral nerves of the upper extremity leading to partial paralysis of the limb; frequently associated with difficult and prolonged labor. **Erb's palsy** results with injury to the upper plexus (C5 and C6), with paralysis of adduction, internal rotation, and pronation. **Klumpke's paralysis** results from injury to the lower plexus (C7, C8, and T1), with paralysis of the muscles of the hand and wrist

bradycardia—slow heart rate; may be associated with apnea during neonatal period

bronchopulmonary dysplasia (BPD)—chronic lung disease secondary to damage to lungs due to mechanical ventilation and oxygen administration in prematurity; predisposes child to frequent upper respiratory infections; effects are usually outgrown after the 1st or 2nd year of life. Places child at increased risk for developmental problems

Broviac—chest catheter for administration of medication

bruxism—grinding of the teeth

bunny hopping—creeping without lower extremity dissociation; both legs move forward together

cerebral palsy (CP)—disorder of posture and movement due to brain damage sustained prenatally, perinatally, or postnatally

choreoathetosis—condition involving involuntary, jerky movements of the extremities

chronological age—child's age since birth

cleft palate—congenital nonfusion deformity of the roof of the mouth leading to an unnatural, open connection between the mouth and nasal cavity

clonus—repetitive, involuntary muscle contractions caused by passive stretch; usually refers to ankle clonus or wrist clonus

clubfoot (see **talipes equinovarus**)

conductive education—training method promoting mobility and activities of daily living skills in people with movement disabilities; initiated in Hungary at the Peto Institute

conductive hearing loss—hearing impairment due to dysfunction in middle ear function

congenital—present at birth; (contrast with genetic and familial)

corrected age—chronological age (in weeks) minus weeks of prematurity

cortical blindness—visual deficit due to damage in the optical areas of the brain; the eyes and visual tracts may be unimpaired

cortical sensory deficit—loss of various sensory abilities due to damage of those areas of the brain, not the sensory organs themselves

coxa plana (Legg-Calve-Perthes disease)—disease process involving aseptic necrosis of the epiphysis of the femoral head; usually unilateral and seen mostly in males; most prevalent between 5–10 years of age

crawl—to move with the arms and legs and with the abdomen on the floor

creep—to move on hands and knees and with the abdomen off of the floor

criterion-referenced—term used to describe assessments that evaluate a child's performance with respect to the attainment of specific criteria rather than compare the child's performance to that of other children the same age

crossing the midline—act of reaching across the body with one extremity

"crouch" posture—standing or walking position characterized by flexion of the lower extremities, with or without trunk flexion

cruise—to walk sideways while holding on to furniture or other supports

cystic fibrosis—genetic disorder of the exocrine glands that is characterized by pulmonary disease, pancreatic enzyme deficiency, and abnormally high sweat electrolytes

cytomegalovirus (CMV)—virus in the herpes family that can cause infection in susceptible individuals; characterized by fever and hepatitis; CMV infection can cause brain damage, vision or hearing loss, and infant death

derotation osteotomy—orthopedic surgical procedure that involves cutting and removing or repositioning of bone to enable proper rotational realignment

developmental delay—chronological delay in any developmental area (speech and language, gross or fine motor, socioemotional, cognitive, etc.)

developmental disability—permanent impairment or handicap in a developmental area that had its origins before adulthood

developmental milestone—behavior or skill typically exhibited at a certain age

developmental sequence—typical progression of developmental milestones

diaphragmatic hernia (hiatus hernia)—protrusion of part of the stomach through the esophageal hiatus of the diaphragm

dissociation—nonsymmetrical positions or actions of 2 parts of the body, especially the extremities and trunk

dorsal rhizotomy (see **selective dorsal rhizotomy**)

Down syndrome—chromosomal abnormality (translocation, mosaicism, or trisomy 21) characterized by certain physical features (especially facial), varying degrees of mental retardation, and hypotonia

ductus arteriosus (see **patent ductus arteriosus**)

dysarthria—articulation disorder due to impairment of the tongue or other muscles involved in speech

dyspnea—labored or difficult breathing

dyspraxia—condition characterized by difficulties with motor planning

dystonia—condition of impaired muscle tone that may result in slow, involuntary motions

early intervention—initiation of developmental services or therapeutic intervention at the earliest indication of potential developmental delay to avoid or minimize potentially permanent or more severe functional impairments

echolalia—repetition of utterances of another person either immediately after they were heard or at a later time; without apparent functional purpose; occurs in typical development, but is considered abnormal when occurring at nontypical ages or if occurring perseveratively

empowerment—process of assisting others in realizing and developing competence and ability to advocate for themselves

endotracheal tube—tube that provides an artificial airway into the trachea

environmental deprivation—disadvantages in a person's living situation that preclude certain opportunities for his or her optimal development

epiphysis—growth plate area of the long bones; ossification site permitting growth in length

equinus—position of plantarflexion

Erb's palsy (see **brachial plexus injury**)

esotropia—turning-in of the eyes

expressive aphasia—inability to speak

extensor thrust—excessive protrusion of the tongue; or, mass extension pattern of the neck, back, or legs

extracorporeal membrane oxygenation (ECMO)—oxygenation of venous blood outside of the body through a gas exchange apparatus in loop with the circulatory system; used in situations of severe, yet reversible, pulmonary or cardiac failure

facilitated communication (FC)—method of assisting people with severe communication disorders to express their needs and feelings through pointing to letters, words, symbols, or through the use of keyboards

facilitation—use of body or joint positions or tactile stimulation to specific muscles to promote muscle activation or the accomplishment of a certain movement

failure to thrive (FTT)—condition characterized by poor weight gain and growth in a child

familial—common occurrence in a family; (contrast with genetic and congenital)

family-centered—philosophy of care that recognizes that a child is an integral part of his or her family, and that the family's needs must be addressed for effective intervention

femoral anteversion—anterior rotation, in the body's transverse plane, of the upper portion of the femur in relation to the femoral condyles; exceeds 25° in infant and young child; decreases to 15° in adult; may cause marked internal rotation of leg if excessive

femoral retroversion—posterior rotation, in the body's transverse plane, of the upper femur in relation to the lower to less than 15° of femoral anteversion; may cause marked external rotation of leg if excessive

fetal alcohol effects (FAE)—term used to indicate that alcohol is being considered as one of the possible causes of a child's birth defects

fetal alcohol syndrome (FAS)—syndrome involving prenatal and/or postnatal growth deficiencies, central nervous system impairment, and characteristic facial morphology; result of maternal alcohol ingestion during pregnancy; minimum necessary dose not yet determined; especially damaging in the 1st trimester

fontanel (or fontanelle)—"soft spot" on an infant's head between unjoined sections of the skull

fragile X syndrome—chromosomal condition that occurs predominantly in males and is characterized by varying degrees of mental retardation, certain physical features such as large head with long face and large ears, increased testicular size, and behavioral features that may include gaze aversion, anxiety, stereotypic movements, and speech difficulties

gastroesophageal reflux (GER or GE reflux)—reflex or back-up of partially ingested food into the esophagus due to insufficient closure of the esophageal sphincter and/or other contributing factors

gastrostomy—small surgical opening through the abdomen into the stomach for direct feeding by means of a tube

gavage feeding—feedings through an oral or nasal tube into the esophagus

genetic—hereditary; transmitted by the genes; may not be manifested at the time of birth, but may appear later in life; (contrast with familial and congenital)

gestational age—infant's age in weeks from 2 weeks prior to mother's last menstrual period before conception to the time of birth; full-term equivalent to 40 weeks

Gower's sign—a way of rising to stand from the floor characterized by the child's "walking up" his or her legs with the hands to gain erect standing; result of proximal muscle weakness; characteristically seen in muscular dystrophy

grand mal seizure (tonic-clonic seizure)—seizure with sudden loss of consciousness, followed by uncontrolled movements of the extremities

gravitational insecurity (postural insecurity)—delayed ability or inability to maintain body segments aligned in space in an antigravity position, especially in response to change of position

Grice procedure—extra-articular arthrodesis of the subtalar joint to stabilize an ankle with surgery

hard palate—bony, anterior roof of the mouth (directly behind the soft palate, teeth)

Harrington rods—metal rods inserted alongside the spine for the treatment of scoliosis; one of several surgical methods used to reduce spinal curvature

heel cup—in-shoe orthotic to improve mild foot malalignment

hernia (see **inguinal, diaphragmatic, or umbilical hernia)**

hiatus hernia (see **diaphragmatic hernia)**

high arched palate—roof of the mouth that is raised more than the norm; may or may not have functional limitations

hippotherapy—use of horseback riding to address specific therapy goals; one of several techniques included in therapeutic horseback riding

human immunodeficiency virus (HIV)—virus that causes infection of and damage to the body's immune system; may also cause encephalopathy and lead to developmental delays; usually acquired in children through medically necessary blood transfusions or transplacentally from an infected mother during pregnancy; some children who test positive at birth may revert to negative by approximately 15 months of age

hyaline membrane disease (HMD) (see **respiratory distress syndrome)**

hydrocephalus—abnormal accumulation of cerebrospinal fluid in the ventricles of the brain; may lead to enlargement of the head and cause brain damage as a result of excessive pressure on the tissues by the fluid

hydromyelia—pooling of cerebrospinal fluid in the central canal in the spinal cord; symptoms may include rapidly developing scoliosis, upper extremity weakness, and increased muscle tone

hyperactivity—excessive behavioral activity level; often associated with attentional deficits

hyperbilirubinemia—condition of excessive bilirubin in the blood; common in neonates; may cause jaundice

IDEA (Individuals with Disabilities Education Act; Public Law 102-119)—federal legislation that describes requirements of educational and early intervention services to children with disabilities. Part B of the Act describes services to children from 3–21 years of age. Part H describes early intervention services provided to children from birth–2 years of age

Ilizarov procedure—procedure to lengthen long bones which utilizes a frame incorporating pins surgically implanted through the bone; pins are separated very slowly (approximately 1mm per day) by elongating the device; promotes bone growth

inclusion—idea of including people with disabilities in regular educational settings, social activities, and any other community program, function, and/or service

Individual Educational Plan (IEP)—written plan of educationally related annual goals (based on the child's/adolescent's specific strengths and needs), objectives, strategies, and timelines to enable the individual between 3–21 years of age to be educated in the least restrictive environment; mandated by law

Individualized Family Service Plan (IFSP)—written plan with specific outcomes and objectives outlining a family's and child's service needs while in early intervention; mandated by law

infantile spasm—seizure characterized by sudden, short, involuntary muscle contractions (usually flexion of the upper extremities and trunk, and extension of the legs) that occurs before 3 years of age

inguinal hernia—protrusion of part of the intestine through the inguinal canal

interdisciplinary—approach involving a group of professionals from various disciplines who collaborate to perform assessments, develop an overall plan of care, and provide intervention to address a child's needs

intonation—changes in the volume or quality of speech

intracranial hemorrhage (ICH)—bleeding inside the skull; can cause neuromotor disorders

intrauterine growth retardation (IUGR) (also see **small for gestational age)**—reduced growth of the fetus in utero that results in birth weight below the 10th percentile for the infant's gestational age

intraventricular hemorrhage (IVH)—bleeding inside the ventricles; can cause neuromotor disorders; 4 grades of IVH: Grades I, II, III, and IV (least to most severe damage); type of intracranial hemorrhage typically associated with prematurity

jargon—unintelligible talk or "nonwords" of a young child; usual aspect of development at certain periods

jaundice—condition caused by the deposition of excess bilirubin in the system and characterized by yellowing of the skin, eyes, mucous membranes, and body fluids

jaw thrust—abnormal jaw movement pattern characterized by strong, downward extension of the mandible often in association with head and neck extensor thrust

juvenile rheumatoid arthritis (JRA)—multiple joint inflammation in children and adolescents that involves swelling, pain, and structural changes; usually affects the large joints with risk of contractures and limitations in function

Klumpke's paralysis (see **brachial plexus injury)**

large for gestational age (LGA)—refers to an infant's weight at birth; encompasses birth weight that is greater than the 90th percentile for the infant's particular gestational age

lateralization—process of developing a dominant preference for one side of the body for functional tasks

learning disability (see **specific learning disability)**

least restrictive environment (LRE)—concept that refers to the right of every child to be educated in as regular an educational environment as possible while still receiving necessary special education or related services

Legg-Calve-Perthes disease (see **coxa plana)**

low birth weight (LBW)—classification indicative of birth weight below 2500 g; very low birth weight (VLBW) includes weights under 1500 g, and extremely low birth weight (ELBW) includes weights under 1000 g

macrocephaly—large head size, with or without hydrocephalus

mainstreaming—process of including children with disabilities in classes with nondisabled children

meconium aspiration—prenatal inhalation of dark, prenatal, fetal, fecal material (meconium); may cause neonatal respiratory compromise

meningocele—birth defect in which there is a protrusion of the meninges through the posterior skull or spinal column; neural tissue not herniated into the protrusion; usually benign

mental retardation—condition characterized by limited intellectual development (IQ under 70) and deficits in adaptive behavior

metatarsus adductus/varus—adduction or varus positioning of the forefeet

microcephaly—small head size; frequently associated with cognitive delay or mental retardation and delayed or impaired development in other areas

midline—theoretical line down the center of the body that separates left from right; corresponds to a sagittal plane bisecting the body

motor planning (see **apraxia**)

M.O.V.E. (Mobility Opportunities Via Education) Program—program utilizing various supportive adaptive equipment to enable children with significant motor involvement to move about their environments with greater independence

multidisciplinary—approach involving several disciplines working distinctly in the assessment, development of an overall plan of care, and provision of intervention to address a child's needs

muscular dystrophy—category of progressive muscular weakness disorders

myelomeningocele—congenital herniations of meninges and neural tissue through an opening at the base of the skull or through the vertebral arches of the spinal cord; associated with paralysis

necrotizing enterocolitis (NEC)—infection of the intestinal tract; frequent in infants born prematurely; may be associated with sepsis

neonatal—concerning an infant's 1st 4–6 weeks of life

nerve block (alcohol block, phenol block)—treatment of spasticity that involves injection of alcohol into nerves of targeted muscles

neurodevelopmental treatment (NDT)—treatment approach emphasizing attainment of antigravity competence for people with neurologically based movement disorders

norm-referenced—term used to describe measurement instruments that compare a child's performance with that of a representative sample of children of same age

nystagmus—involuntary, rapid eye movements

object permanence—awareness of an object's existence after it has been removed from the visual field; child can find it in a hidden location

omphalocele (see **umbilical hernia**)

opisthotonus—mass involuntary extension (posterior curvation) of the body

opposition—movement of the thumb toward the palm or fingers

Ortolani (reduction) test—test for hip dislocation; a "clunk" is felt/heard upon movement of the femoral head back onto the acetabulum while the thigh is in abduction and flexion

Osgood-Schlatter's disease—disease process involving osteochondritis of the tibial tubercle; more common in boys; most prevalent between 10–15 years of age

osteogenesis imperfecta ("brittle bone disease")—inherited disorder of cartilage formation that is characterized by excessive fragility of bones and is associated with frequent fractures

osteotomy—cutting of a bone in a surgical procedure (for realignment)

otitis media—middle ear infection

patent ductus arteriosus (PDA)—persistent fetal circulation due to failure of the opening between the aorta and the main pulmonary artery to close shortly after birth; may require chemical or surgical ligation if it does not close

perceptual-motor dysfunction—dysfunction characterized by the inability to integrate (take in, organize, and synthesize) particular types of perceptual and sensory stimuli to support functional motor output

periventricular leukomalacia (PVL)—necrosis of white matter adjacent to the ventricles of the brain as a result of ischemia; often associated with prematurity and Grades III and IV intraventricular hemorrhage; may result in cerebral palsy

perseveration—repetitive continuation of an action (motor, speech, or mental); may be normal during certain learning processes or, if inappropriate, may be pathological

pervasive developmental disorder (PDD)—developmental disability characterized by qualitative impairment in reciprocal social interaction and verbal and nonverbal communication skills; repertoire of activities may be restricted

petit mal seizure (see **absence seizure**)

phenol block (see **nerve block**)

phonation—production of voiced sound by means of vocal cord vibrations

phototherapy—use of specialized lights for the treatment of hyperbilirubinimia, typically for newborn infants

physiological flexion—flexion bias seen in the normal, full-term neonate associated with intrauterine confinement

postrotary nystagmus—reflexive oscillatory movements of the eyes after rotational stimulation such as spinning; should cease after a few seconds

postural control—graded, coordinated muscle control to providing appropriate posture for a specific task

postural insecurity (see **gravitational insecurity**)

praxis (motor planning)—ability to perform sequenced, coordinated movement in relation to functional demands

prehension—grasp

premature rupture of membranes (PROM)—early rupture of membranes surrounding the fetus; precipitates birth and is a cause of premature birth

preterm—refers to birth of child before 37 weeks' gestation; preferable to term "premature"

raking—moving of small objects with the whole hand, using the fingers against the palm without inclusion of the thumb

receptive aphasia—inability to understand or act upon spoken language

regulatory disorder—disorder characterized by significant problems in the domains of sleep, self-consoling, feeding, transitions, and distress at caregiving and play experiences involving sensory challenges

respiratory syntitial virus (RSV)—virus that causes acute lower respiratory disease (such as pneumonia) and can be fatal in severe cases

respiratory distress syndrome (RDS, hyaline membrane disease)—respiratory distress due to atelectasis caused by insufficient surfactant in premature lungs; may lead to acute respiratory failure and death; chronic RDS and mechanical ventilation often contribute to bronchopulmonary dysplasia (BPD)

retinopathy of prematurity (ROP)—condition involving damage to the eyes during the neonatal period due to abnormal growth of blood vessels; thought to be related to supplemental oxygen administration; various classifications exist (levels I–IV) from minimal impairment to complete blindness as a result of complete retinal detachment

reverse last shoes—shoes that look as if the right were actually the left shoe and vice versa; may be used in the treatment of metatarsus adductovarus

rhizotomy (see **selective dorsal rhizotomy**)

sacral sitting—kyphotic sitting position characterized by weightbearing on the sacrum rather than on the ischial tuberosities

scissoring—adduction or crossing of 1 leg over the other during standing and stepping; associated with adductor spasticity

selective dorsal (or posterior) rhizotomy—surgical technique involving the cutting of selected dorsal roots to reduce spasticity that interferes with muscular control and function; same objective may be achieved temporarily with use of baclofen pump or spinal cord stimulation

self-stimulation—abnormal, excessive, or inappropriate behaviors exhibited by a person with sensory deficits to supplement sensory experiences; often seen in individuals with severe cognitive deficit, autism, and related disorders

sensorineural hearing loss—hearing impairment due to neurological (inner ear and/or auditory nerve) rather than structural (conductive) reasons

sensory integration—reception, organization, and synthesis of sensory and environmental stimuli to support appropriate motor responses

sensory integration therapy—treatment approach for individuals with sensory integration dysfunctions; use of vestibular, proprioceptive, and tactile stimulation interventions to promote improved processing of sensory information for adaptive responses to environmental demands

serial casting—process of recasting a limb with several successive casts (each usually worn for 1 week) to improve range of motion of a particular joint through soft tissue elongation

service coordinator—person responsible for the organization of all services (early intervention, medical, and social) to address needs of a child and his or her family under an IFSP

shunt—tube that is implanted to drain excess fluid from the brain to the peritoneal cavity; children with spina bifida and hydrocephalus frequently have ventriculi-peritoneal (VP) shunts; shunt malfunction warning signs include vomiting, irritability, loss of appetite, increased muscle tone, drowsiness/lethargy, seizures, and swelling along the shunt

slipped capital (femoral) epiphysis—displacement of the proximal femoral epiphysis associated with pain and external rotation positioning; condition is usually unilateral; occurs primarily in 10–17 year-olds; more common in males

small for gestational age (SGA) (see **intrauterine growth retardation**)—birth weight that is below the 10th percentile for the infant's particular gestational age

soft palate (velum)—soft muscular sheath attached to the posterior portion of the hard palate which helps separate the nasal cavity from the oral cavity

specific learning disability (SLD)—term used for any of a group of disabilities characterized by difficulties in understanding, using, or perceiving language, vision or movement because of processing difficulties that are not the result of mental retardation or other identifiable impairments; affects school performance

spica cast—cast extending from mid torso to below knee used to address hip dislocation or, fractures used during postsurgery to hold femur in acetabula with the thighs in a position of abduction and external rotation

spina bifida—congenital malformation of vertebral arches; often associated with neural tube defects such as myelomeningocele; degree of disability depends on spinal levels involved

strabismus—optical disorder involving misalignment of one or both eyes; esotropia, exotropia are examples of strabismus

straight last shoes—shoes with a neutral last that can be worn on the right or left foot; used in treating mild forefoot alignment problems

subtalar neutral (STN)—position of the subtalar joint where it is neither supinated nor pronated; calcaneus is perpendicular to the ground and aligned with distal 1/3 of leg

subtalar valgus—position of the subtalar joint where the heel is turned out relative to the structures above it; also called cancaneal eversion or hindfoot eversion

subtalar varus—position of the subtalar joint where the heel is turned in

sudden infant death syndrome (SIDS)—term used in the unexpected death of an infant for which a pathological cause cannot be determined; evidence increasing for relationship with prone sleeping

surfactant—lung substance that prevents alveolar collapse by maintaining surface tension within the alveoli; begins to be produced at approximately 24 weeks' gestational age and reaches a critical value at approximately 32 weeks' gestational age

tachycardia—increased heart rate

tachypnea—increased respiratory rate

talipes equinovarus (clubfoot)—deformity of the foot/ankle complex involving plantarflexion, inversion, adduction, and possible associated cavus deformity

tandem walking—walking on a straight line, placing heel of 1 foot in front of the toes of the other at each step

teratogenic—environmental substances or factors which can cause congenital deformities or conditions

tethered cord—adhesion of the spinal cord within the spinal canal with successive shredding and/or damage due to stretching of the structures with growth; frequently associated with spina bifida, especially myelomeningocele; causes a deterioration of previous skills; requires surgical repair

tetralogy of Fallot—cardiac condition involving 4 defects: pulmonary stenosis, ventricular septal defect, overriding aorta, and right ventricular hypertrophy

tibial torsion—spiraling of the tibia common in newborn infants; affects lower extremity alignment and gait, if excessive; distinguish from rotation of the tibia at the knee, relative to the femur

tongue thrust—abnormally forceful protrusion of the tongue

tongue lateralization—movement of the tongue to the sides of the mouth in order to position foods between the teeth for chewing

tonic-clonic seizure (see **grand mal seizure**)

total communication—communication approach involving use of verbal and nonverbal communication techniques

tracheostomy—surgical opening in the throat to provide an alternate airway

tracking—moving the eyes to follow an object moving through the visual field

transdisciplinary—team approach in which members from various disciplines work together and cross traditional discipline boundaries for comprehensive assessment, development of a care plan, and intervention to address a child's needs

transition—process of moving from 1 position to another (from sitting to standing) or from one care setting to another (from hospital to an early intervention program)

tympanogram—diagnostic procedure for the examination of the eustachian tubes and middle ear

umbilical hernia (omphalocele)—defect in the abdominal wall allowing protrusion around the navel; often subsides without intervention

ventricular septal defect (VSD)—abnormal opening between the cardiac ventricles

W-sitting—sitting in a wide kneeling position with the bottom in contact with the ground between the legs; displayed by average children; only abnormal when it is the child's only means of independently achieved sitting; puts internal rotational stresses on the hip joint, medial stresses on knee structures, and plantarflexion/inversion stresses on the foot/ankle complex

Wilms' tumor—a childhood cancer that originates in the kidneys; found predominantly in children from infant–15 years of age, with diagnosis usually by 5 years of age; can be fatal if not identified and treated aggressively

Figure/Table Credits

FIGURES

Figure 2.1. Adapted from Gilfoyle EM, ed. Training: occupational therapy education management in schools. Rockville, MD: American Occupational Therapy Association, 1981.
Figure 2.2. Adapted from Wong DL, Whaley LF. Nursing care of infant and children, 3rd ed. St. Louis: CV Mosby, 1990:1088.
Figure 2.3. Reproduced from Shumway-Cook A, Horak FB. Assessing the influence of sensory interaction on balance. Physical Therapy 1986; 1548–1550.
Figure 2.4. & 2.5. From Campbell PH. Evaluation and assessment in early intervention for infants and toddlers. Journal of Early Intervention 1991;15:36–45.
Figures 4.1 and 4.4. From TherAdapt Products, Inc., Bensenville, IL.
Figures 4.2, 4.3, 4.5, & 4.7. From Rifton, Rifton, NY.
Figures 4.6 and 4.8. From Kaye Products, Inc., Hillsborough, NC.
Figures 4.9–4.21. From Southpaw Enterprises, Inc., Dayton, OH.

TABLES

Table 1.1. From Harris SR, Tada WL. Genetic disorders. In: Umphred DA, ed. Neurological rehabilitation. St. Louis: CV Mosby, 1990: 258 –281; Moore KL, Persaud TVN. The developing human, 5th ed. Philadelphia: WB Saunders, 1993:14–39, 142–173.
Table 1.2. Adapted from Villarreal SF, McKinney L, Quackenbush M. Handle with care: helping children prenatally wxposed to drugs and alcohol. Santa Cruz, CA: ETR Associates, 1992:172–176
Table 1.3–1.5. From Bacon GE, Spenser ML, Hopwood NJ, Kelch RP. Pediatric endocrinology. Chicago: Year Book, 1990;62–122; Graham JM. Smith's recognizable pattern of human deformation, 2nd ed. Philadelphia: WB Saunders, 1988; Jones KL. Smith's recognizable pattern of human malformation, 4th ed. Philadelphia: WB Saunders, 1988
Table 1.6–1.8. Adapted from Hensinger RN. Standards in pediatric orthopedics. New York: Raven Press, 1986:49, 53, 251.
Table 1.10. Beckoff A. Embryonic motor output and movement patterns: relationship to postnatal behavior. In: Smotherman WP, Robinson SR, eds. Behavior of the fetus. Caldwell, NJ: Telfrod Press, 1988:191–206; Folio MR, Fewell RR. Peabody Development Motor Scales. Hingham, MA: Teaching Resources Corp., 1983; Bottos M, Dalla Barba B, Stephani D, et al. locomotor strategies preceding independent walking: prospective study of neurological and language development in 42 cases. Developmental Medicine and Child Neurology 1989;31:25–34.
Table 1.11. Folio MR, Fewell RR. Peabody Developmental Motor Scales. Hingham, MA: Teaching Resources Corp., 1983; Bruininks RH. Bruininks-Oretsky Test of Motor Proficiency. Circle Pines, MN: American Guidance Service, 1978.
Table 2.1. Adapted from Dunn W. Pediatric occupational therapy: facilitating effective service provision. Thorofare, NJ: Slack, Inc. 1991:43.
Table 2.4. Adapted from Cintas H, Scull S. APTA Combined Section Meeting, 1985.
Table 2.5. From Harris MB, Simons CJ, Ritchie SK, Mullett MD, Myerberg DZ. Joint range of motion development in premature infants. Pediatric Physical Therapy 1990;2:185–192.
Table 2.6. From Wilson JM, Cerebral palsy. IN: Campbell SK, ed. Pediatric neurologic physical therapy. New York: Churchill Livingstone, 1991; 215–249.
Table 2.7. From Blaskey J. Head trauma. In: Campbell SK, ed. Pediatric neurologic physical therapy. New York: Churchill Livingstone, 1991; 215–249.
Table 2.8. From Donohue B, Turner D, Worrell T. The use of functional reach as a measurement of balance in typically developing boys and girls ages 5-15 years. Pediatric Physical Therapy 1994;6: 189–193
Table 2.9. From Heriza CB. Kinematic motion analysis. In: Wilhelm IJ, ed. Physical therapy assessment in early infancy. New York: Churchill Livingstone, 1993; 257–292.

Tables 2.10 & 2.11. From Gould A. Cardiopulmonary evaluation of the infant, toddler, child and adolescent. Pediatric Physical Therapy 1991; 3 (11): 9–13.

Table 2.12. Adapted from American Heart Association Report: Standards for exercise testing in the pediatric age group. In: Oded Bar-Or. Pediatric sports medicine for the practitioner. New York: Springer-Verlag, 1983.

Table 3.2. Allsop K. Muscular dystrophy, spinal muscle atrophy, and related disorders. In: Payton OD, ed. Manual of physical therapy. New York: Churchill Livingstone, 1989; 309–325. Cumming WJK. Neuromuscular disorders. In: Eckersley PM, ed. Elements of paediatric disorders. Edinburgh: Churchill Livingstone, 1993; 187–201.

Table 5.1. Beck RJ, Andriacci TP, Kuo KN et al. Changes in the gait patterns of growing children. Journal of Bone and Joint Surgery 1981; 63A:1452–1456. Kucera M, Macek M, Javurek J. A method for estimation of the changes in bipedal locomotion. In: Berg K, Eriksson BO, eds. Children and exercise IX. 1980; 49–52. Sutherland DH, Olshen RA, Biden EN, Wyatt MP. The development of mature walking. Clinics in Development Medicine No. 104/105. London: Mac Keith Press, 1988.

Table 5.2. Gage JR. Gait analysis in cerebral palsy. Clinics in Development Medicine No. 121. London: Mac Keith Press, 1991. Sutherland DH, Valencia F. Pediatric gait: normal and abnormal development. In: Drennen JC, ed. The child's foot and ankle. New York: Raven, 1992; 19–35. Wenger DR, Rang M. The art and practice of children's orthopedics. New York: Raven, 1993.

Table 5.3. Rose J, Gamble JG. Human Walking. 2nd ed. Baltimore: Williams & Wilkins, 1994. Whittle MW. Gait analysis: an introduction. Oxford: Butterworth-Heinemann, 1991. Winter DA. Biomechanics of human movement. New York: Wiley, 1979.

Table 6.1. Adapted from Smith BJ, Rose DF, Ballard JB, Walsh S. The preschool (Part B) and infant, toddler (Part H) program of the Individuals with Disabilities Education Act (IDEA) and the 1991 amendments (PL 1-2–119): selected comparisons.

Table 6.2. From Woodruff A, McGonigel MI. Early intervention team approaches: the transdisciplinary model. In: Jordan JB, Gallagher JJ, Hutinger PL, Karnes MB, eds. Early childhood special education: birth to three. Reston, VA: Council for Exceptional Children, 1988; 166.

Table 6.3. From Long T, Raver SA. Neuromotor development in infants and young children. In: Raver SA, ed. Strategies for teaching at-risk and handicapped infants and toddlers: a transdisciplinary approach. New York: MacMillan, 1991; 48.

Table 6.6. From Section on Pediatrics. Physical therapy practice in educational environments. Alexandria, VA: American Physical Therapy Association, 1990; 7:7.

Index

Page numbers in *italics* denote figures; those followed by "t" denote tables.